Alzheimer's, Aromatherapy,
and the
Sense of Smell

"*Alzheimer's, Aromatherapy, and the Sense of Smell* thoroughly decodes and describes Alzheimer's disease, its complexities, potential causes, consequences, and considerations. Relating to current research and personal and professional experience, Jean-Pierre Willem presents a clear, easy-to-assimilate holistic overview of this debilitating condition in a way that is honest, enlightening, and especially hopeful, revealing both supportive and preventive strategies to proactively engage. As well as exploring the associated cognitive and emotional virtues of familiar essential oils, such as rosemary, lavender, and frankincense, Jean-Pierre also introduces less commonly known exotic oils that are native to Madagascar—such as butterfly ginger, grains of paradise, and herbe des rois (herb of kings)—to provide an invaluable repertoire of useful essential oils and synergistic blends. This timely book is a valuable resource, not only for those affected by Alzheimer's disease but also for anyone interested in maintaining their cognitive alertness, function, and well-being."

HEATHER DAWN GODFREY P.G.C.E., B.SC. AUTHOR OF
HEALING WITH ESSENTIAL OILS

Alzheimer's, Aromatherapy,
and the
Sense of Smell

Essential Oils to
Prevent Cognitive Loss
and Restore Memory

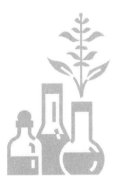

JEAN-PIERRE WILLEM, M.D.
TRANSLATED BY JON E. GRAHAM

Healing Arts Press
Rochester, Vermont

Healing Arts Press
One Park Street
Rochester, Vermont 05767
www.HealingArtsPress.com

Text stock is SFI certified

Healing Arts Press is a division of Inner Traditions International

Originally published in French under the title *Alzheimer & odorat: Quand les arômes restaurent la mémoire: Une piste pour le traitement* by Guy Trédaniel éditeur
First U.S. edition published in 2022 by Healing Arts Press

Note to the reader: *This book is intended as an informational guide. The remedies, approaches, and techniques described herein are meant to supplement, and not to be a substitute for, professional medical care or treatment. They should not be used to treat a serious ailment without prior consultation with a qualified health care professional.*

Cataloging-in-Publication Data for this title is available from the Library of Congress

ISBN 978-1-64411-443-8 (print)
ISBN 978-1-64411-444-5 (ebook)

Printed and bound in the United States by Lake Book Manufacturing, Inc. The text stock is SFI certified. The Sustainable Forestry Initiative® program promotes sustainable forest management.

10 9 8 7 6 5 4 3 2 1

Text design and layout by Virginia Scott Bowman
This book was typeset in Garamond Premier Pro with Minion Pro and Architecta used as the display typefaces

Contents

INTRODUCTION

Understanding Alzheimer's 1

1 **Alzheimer's Disease Decoded** 7
Evolution of the Human
Olfactory System

2 **Cerebral Lesions and
Their Consequences** 14
A Look inside the Anomalies
of the Alzheimer's Brain

3 **How to Establish the Diagnosis** 22
A Multidisciplinary Approach

4 **Laboratory Analysis** 40
Biochemical Factors for Diagnosis, Prevention,
and Treatment

5 **The Brain and Its Neurons** 51
A Primer

6 **A Stroll Down Memory Lane** 61
The Systems and Stages of Memory

7 **Development of the Disease** 69
The Stages and Progression of Alzheimer's

8 The Multiple Causes of Alzheimer's Disease 81
Medications, Mitochondria, and More

9 Additional Risk Factors and Considerations 96
Knowledge Is Power

10 The Body's Five Protective Barriers 112
And What Happens When They Rupture

11 Neuroplasticity 123
Caring for the Brain

12 Alzheimer's Disease and the Sense of Smell 133
A Closer Look at Our Primary Sense

13 Finding Help from Essential Oils 141
The Benefits and Practice of Olfactory Therapy

14 The Cooking of Food 163
Problems and Solutions

15 Return to the Raw 171
Establishing an Olfactory-Friendly Diet

16 Prevention 179
Tips for Maintaining a Healthy Mental State

17 We Are What We Eat 185
Brain Food Supplements

18 Navigating Alzheimer's Disease 205
A Guide for Families and Caregivers

CONCLUSION

Writing a New Page of Medical History   214

APPENDIX 1

Diseases Akin to Alzheimer's   219

APPENDIX 2

The Nose Knows   228
Learning from Man's Best Friend

Bibliography   236

Index   240

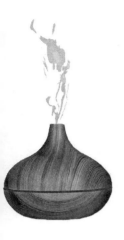

Understanding Alzheimer's

ALZHEIMER'S DISEASE is one of the major public health problems of the United States and Europe, as it is in all the countries of the developed world. The Alzheimer's Association estimated that six million Americans were living with Alzheimer's in 2021, and at the current pace, if there are no improvements in treatment or prevention, that number is projected to climb to almost thirteen million by 2050.

These impressive figures give an idea of the effect Alzheimer's and similar disorders are having on the American population, especially given that human beings are living longer and longer. It comes as no surprise that under these conditions, most of us fear growing old because we associate aging with the loss of memory, the loss of reason, and all too often the loss of our dignity.

The disease is quite insidious in the beginning. After about the age of fifty, many people begin to experience memory lapses: they forget people's names, they can't remember where they set down their eyeglasses, they forget to make a call they had promised to make. For most of us, these events remain trivial and are of no consequence. For a small number of individuals, these anomalies are accompanied by more disturbing changes: their notion of time grows fuzzy, spaces seem foreign to them, they no longer recognize their everyday surroundings, and after a while the actions of daily life become more challenging. After a long and sometimes pitfall-strewn path, the verdict comes in: they are suffering from Alzheimer's disease. Gradually the ravages of the cognitive functions alter their behavior. Their ability to relate to other people changes, which becomes a source of misunderstanding and pain both for the patients and their families.

We do, of course, have tremendous need for information about how to understand and act in a way that can help Alzheimer's patients. But the figures don't speak to the suffering and hardship incurred by living with this disease for many years—or the suffering and hardship experienced by those who are close to a patient.

Alzheimer's disease is caused by cerebral alterations. It is therefore a brain disease. But it is more than that.

It is a personality disorder because it alters the mental function of a loved one by changing their intellectual functions as well as their emotional life.

It is a family disorder, because your loved one becomes a different person and his or her relationship with you changes. More or less quickly, the entire family is immersed, despite all, in the many problems caused by keeping the affected person at home. The demands on morale and people's physical abilities become a source of stress, anxiety, and depression.

It is also a social disease, because, as a disease connected with aging, its frequency will only increase with the lengthening life expectancy of an aging population. This phenomenon creates social problems that go far beyond the purely medical aspect of the disease.

THE CURRENT STATE OF RESEARCH

At the current time, Alzheimer's is the most common form of dementia in the industrialized world and, according to the World Health Organization, one of the top ten leading causes of death. So it should come as no surprise that research in this field is particularly intense.

What might come as a surprise, on the other hand, is that the majority of theories are based on the idea of a single causative factor, one maintained by experts who have made it the cornerstone of their careers. These opinion leaders will not tolerate any explanation capable of challenging their theories.

The most common theory is oriented toward the aggregation of beta-amyloid, a kind of protein primarily found in the brain, which becomes toxic when it accumulates and combines. But beta-amyloids only accumulate in the brain over the course of many years in an inflamed terrain. So, some authors mention a very promising theory of inflammation as an avenue for brain degeneration. Others believe that eliminating all risk factors will solve the problem. Olivier Saint-Jean, head of the geriatric department of the Georges Pompidou European Hospital in Paris, created a horde of enemies by labeling Alzheimer's disease as a "social construct"—a pathologizing of the common occurrence of cognitive decline in the elderly.

There are stacks of books on this subject in bookstores. In them we find the same ingredients for overcoming this infernal disease: eliminate environmental pollutants and plug up the nutritional deficiencies that come about, especially in the final stages of decline. But there's nothing original here, as this same approach is recommended for every pathological condition.

In June 2014, the largest congress in the world on Alzheimer's brought some 4,500 experts together in Copenhagen, and they came to this conclusion: "The major problem for the development of promising new methods of treatment is that research has yet to identify with certainty the molecular mechanisms that trigger this disease."

Essentially, as the members of that congress implied, what we are looking for are the molecular mechanisms that would make it possible to develop an effective treatment. However, Alzheimer's is like a jigsaw puzzle made up of jagged pieces. Instead of putting these pieces together, researchers spend their time isolating and analyzing the puzzle piece that looks the most promising to them. The puzzle as a whole, then, remains a brainteaser. If we continue to pursue this path, we will never put the puzzle together, and the problem will remain insoluble.

Other paths are open to us. For example, neurologist Dale Bredesen has oriented his research around the idea that Alzeheimer's is a multifactorial disease and declining cognitive function can be restored thanks to an intensive multifactorial program. In *The End of Alzheimer's,* Bredesen explains that the existing medications for treating Alzheimer's only concentrate on one aspect, but that path is ineffective because Alzheimer's disease is complex. To illustrate his theory, he resorts to a metaphor that goes something like this: Imagine that you have a roof with thirty-six holes in it. You call roofers for help, and they come and patch one of the holes. So now that one hole is no longer a problem, but thirty-five holes still remain, letting in the rain, and inside your house the situation has not really changed. That, Bredesen says, is the problem with Alzheimer's research and treatments. If the disease has multiple causes, treatments designed to address one specific cause won't help.

Bredesen uses the metaphor of thirty-six holes in the roof because he believes that Alzheimer's can be caused by at least thirty-six factors. These factors can be determined by a battery of medical exams that divide patients into three primary categories of causation: inflammatory (chronic inflammation), atrophic (deficiency of hormones or vitamins), or toxic (presence of toxic substances). Once the risk factors are identified, an individualized care protocol can be designed for the patient.

While Bredesen's approach is certainly interesting, his critics claim that he pushes an aggressive and perhaps self-serving intervention, even with patients who are starting to experience a cognitive decline that has not been clearly identified as dementia, never mind Alzheimer's, and without any control group. His results do show that lifestyle changes can slow the onset or aggravation of symptoms, but much remains uncertain at this stage. Furthermore, patients would need to follow Bredesen's treatment protocol for the rest of their lives, which, given the cost of the treatment, makes for a thriving business opportunity and raises skepticism.

REORIENTING THE SEARCH

When we find ourselves at an impasse, the sole possible solution is to radically change direction while rigorously setting aside dogmas that have become outdated and considering all the scientific facts from a new angle. In this case, our new perspective can include the insights offered by the science of paleoanthropology. Research into the history of human evolution shows that our taste for modernization and what we believe is an improved lifestyle inspires us to live in conformance with the laws of the market rather than those of our species. Little by little, we draw ever further away from demands of the body that are genetically anchored in us.

With the complex, vicious cycles that dominate the development of Alzheimer's disease, it is essential to take a systemic approach, on a biological level, as advocated by Hippocrates some 2,400 years ago. With so much of Alzheimer's research to date focused on finding a single medication—a miracle cure—that is capable of stopping this disease, we have overlooked consideration of a nonmedicinal solution based on a systemic approach to the problem.

THE OLFACTORY SYSTEM, THE PROVIDENTIAL SENSE

Something to deplore is that researchers have not lingered over the various clinical signs exhibited by those patients afflicted by cognitive problems and other behavioral disorders. One of the very first signs, and one that is omnipresent, is changes in the olfactory sense, the most sophisticated of the five senses. Not coincidentally, the olfactory system is connected to our limbic brain, which contains our hippocampus and amygdala, the keys to memory and emotion. Perhaps, as we'll discuss throughout this book, restoration of the olfactory system through the use of aromatherapy, together with the restoration of the entire body through a living diet focused on raw foods, can be the systemic approach for which we have been looking.

Active support of this research remains one of the obvious keys to progress in the prevention and treatment of this terrifying disease.

The development of an Alzheimer's disease prevention policy will be a major stake in the years to come. For this reason, it is essential to know and master the factors that can hinder cognitive decline linked to aging and the onset of Alzheimer's. This will involve clinical trials on the general population, some of which have already been initiated and have shown promise in England, Germany, Japan, China, and France, especially in senior living facilities.

Alzheimer's is no longer the inevitable destiny for people growing older. A book like this is a direct emission from the breach presently opened in the ocean of indifference in which, until now, were drowning individuals whose aging could not unfurl as it should: in peace, the serenity of a long journey fulfilled, and the happiness of another life with . . . a few more years.

> *If someone desires health, he must be asked if he is ready to remove the causes of his illness.*
>
> HIPPOCRATES, 460–377 BCE

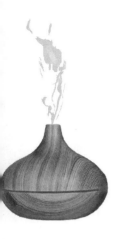

1

Alzheimer's Disease Decoded

Evolution of the Human Olfactory System

SOME DISCOVERIES are made by chance or intuition, but the majority come from observations. In terms of Alzheimer's, with its rich symptomatology, one particular clinical observation can suffice for diagnosis and should orient the direction taken by researchers: anosmia. In fact, 95 percent of people suffering from Alzheimer's disease are affected by the loss of their sense of smell.

No longer being able to smell the odors of nature, of those close to you, or of a perfume, no longer being able to enjoy the flavors of a dish—all these olfactory deficiencies have an undeniably adverse effect on a person's quality of life. For clinical purposes, loss of the sense of smell comes into play in the very first stages of the disease. However, it can be difficult to evaluate this sensorial deficit because the majority of the tests used require, in addition to sensorial and perceptual capacities, cognitive abilities and an attention span, all of which tend to become dulled with age, even when no dementia is present.

Many studies have shown that patients with a genetic risk of Alzheimer's disease or those who have moderate cognitive impairment exhibit significantly greater olfactory alterations than healthy individuals. Conversely, many other studies have shown that people who present with anosmia (complete loss of smell) or hyposmia (reduced sense of smell) are more likely to develop dementia than people who retain their sense of smell.

This specific impairment of the olfactory system in Alzheimer's disease, as well as its connection with the limbic system and the strong emotional power of olfactory memory, make a powerful argument for directing our attention toward the effect of olfactory disorders in this disease.

EMPLOYING PALEONTOLOGY

When we study phylogenesis—namely, the historical evolution of the human species—we learn that our ancestors went through two major epochs: that of the raw, in which the olfactory system dominated, and then, after the discovery of fire, that of the cooked, in which the gustatory system became dominant.

Throughout evolution, every living species, particularly *Homo sapiens,* created defense systems in response to hostile surroundings. These genetically determined mechanisms are specific to species sharing the same biotope. One adapts to one's environment and to one's hostile neighbors to survive. Our ancient ancestors used their olfactory system (their sense of smell) as a compass to guide their survival instincts.

First Epoch: The Raw

In the beginning, there was the primitive diet, an "animal" type of diet that was raw and intended to ensure the essentials—namely, survival, reproduction, and adaptation. This raw diet was guided by the olfactory system. As Dr. Félix Affoyon, who has been studying the mechanisms of Alzheimer's disease, notes:

It is likely not by chance that, over the course of evolution, the regions of the cerebral cortex that retained a connection with the olfactory system are the phylogenetically speaking ancient systems, such as the hippocampus of the limbic brain, which we know plays a fundamental role in the acquisition of memory, learning, and the emotional aspects of behavior, and the amygdala, which is involved in the emotions and emotional learning. It so happens that these regions are the ones that are affected in Alzheimer's disease. (Affoyon 2010)

In other words, our ancestors' sense of smell guided their behavior, cognitive skills, and development.

Second Epoch: The Cooked

With the advent of cooking, humans began to face the intrusion of antigens, substances that our cells recognized as foreign and aggressive. Some paleoanthropologists maintain that this happened 20,000 years ago, in the Neolithic period, when our ancestors transitioned from hunter-gatherers to food producers. Over the course of the millennia and under the repeated assault of the foreign molecules introduced by high-temperature cooking, the olfactory system, which was our primary warning system for the presence of danger, underwent considerable genetic mutations until, slowly but surely, our ancestors' primitive instinct for survival, reproduction, and adaptation eroded. As Dr. Affoyon notes:

If, today, human beings are no longer capable of trusting their sense of smell as they once did to avoid toxic foods and foreign molecules, it is because they altered, by chance, the course of things by discovering cooking, the transformation and preservation of foods, which over the course of evolution developed the sense of taste, gradually relegating the sense of smell to a vestigial state. (Affoyon 2010)

Cooking food did some of the same work that our ancestors had previously relied on their sense of smell to do, helping them avoid pathogens (by killing them) and certain toxins (by deactivating them). Unfortunately, it also reduced certain enzymatic processes that our bodies rely on to process raw foods, and it did not necessarily neutralize the full toxic arsenal found in food. Quite the contrary, for our bodies have a second filter: the intestinal immune barrier, in which wait the cells whose purpose is to detect even the smallest antigen and neutralize it. As the human species adapted over time, our increasing reliance on that antigen immune response went hand in hand with a decreasing use of the olfactory and limbic systems.

This is how over the course of the millennia a cooked diet (enjoyed no longer by smell but by taste) has produced a gradual decline and involution of the olfactory system and an inhibition of the physiological functions of the sense of smell, the hippocampus, and the limbic system. To restore our olfactory function, and the memory and emotion structures and processes connected to it, it is necessary to reverse direction.

There are two approaches available to us for restoring the olfactory system: returning to a living-food diet and stimulating the olfactory system with essential oils.

RETURNING TO A LIVING-FOOD DIET

Eating raw food is one answer to current dietary shifts, a way of healthy nutrition that reconciles pleasure and health. All the animals alive on this planet, in their natural diet, feed exclusively on raw foods. We humans are the only species that cook our food—and we are among the few that are stricken by degenerative diseases, a fate also suffered by the domestic animals that share our ecosystem.

Gandhi said that to get rid of a disease, it is necessary to eliminate the use of fire in the preparation of meals.

Today, the virtues and pertinence of a primarily plant-based diet, one that is mostly raw, unprocessed, organic or biodynamic, and preferably grown locally, are increasingly recognized by health and nutrition specialists as well as the public at large. There are still hindrances to a return to this kind of diet, mainly activated by the powerful players of corporate agriculture, agro-chemistry, and large-scale animal raising. Nevertheless, the principles and foods that govern and make up the concept of a living diet have become increasingly integrated into our lifestyles. They occupy growing space on the shelves of supermarkets and specialty stores alike.

A living diet pursues the goal of giving our bodies foods that offer high nutritional density, are closest to their natural state, and are easy for our bodies to assimilate. For this reason, these foods have to be plant based and mostly raw and organic. Among the countless possibilities, several hold an important place: sprouted grains, freshwater microalgae, seaweed, freshly extracted fruit and vegetable juices, so-called green juices made from wheatgrass and young sprouts, oleaginous fruits and seeds, and fresh fruits and vegetables that are in season and locally produced.

These living foods, which are essentially those high in chlorophyll, and therefore have high enzyme and oxygen content, represent the purest, most original, and most concentrated source of nutritive elements. Chlorophyll is the green pigment characteristic of the majority of plants. It is the primary vector of the life cycle because it plays a role in photosynthesis. Without chlorophyll, there would be no life on planet Earth— no plants, no animals, and no human beings. In other words, the health of the human being, who is at the top of the food chain, and that of the planet are intrinsically connected. From soil to plate, all the stages share equal importance. The essential secret of a living-food diet precisely resides in this integrative or global approach to our food.

Obviously, it is not possible to eat a 100 percent raw diet. Some raw foods, like potatoes, beans, and grains, are indigestible and can be made digestible and flavorful only through cooking. This is why I recommend following a diet that is 70 percent raw food and 30 percent cooked food.

All vitamins in their natural (raw) state are recognizable to our bodies and easily metabolized. The colloidal state of the cell in raw food is specific to its living status; cooking destroys it.

STIMULATING THE SENSE OF SMELL WITH ESSENTIAL OILS

Alzheimer's disease is an important field of research in relation to aromatherapy. Numerous studies already exist that reveal the value of essential oils for treating this pathological condition. For example, in Japan researchers have observed that the diffusion of rosemary and lemon essential oils in the morning and a blend of lavender and neroli essential oils at night restores the olfactory system in elderly people after a period of twenty-eight days. Alzheimer's patients in this study saw improvement in cognitive function, including abstract thinking, and slight improvement in motor skills (Jimbo et al. 2009).

Essential Oils and the Neurosciences

Inhaling essential oils alters our cerebral activity. Many studies have shown that different compounds in essential oils have varying effects on, for example, alpha and beta wave activity, as measured by electroencephalogram (EEG). Some essential oils have stimulating effects, others have relaxing effects, and still others have different effects. But while the physiological effects of aromatic essential oils have been the subject of much research on topics ranging from brain activity to blood pressure and cardiac rhythm, the more subtle effect of odors on our minds are just beginning to be mapped out.

In Garches, France, essential oil specialists are leading workshops in the rehabilitation department of the Raymond Poincaré University Hospital. Their objective: stimulating individuals who have been victims of a stroke by having them smell a variety of common everyday odors such as cookies, toast, candy, and freshly cut grass. "Through a direct connection to the memory, the patients have managed, thanks to aromas, to re-appropriate a portion of their personal histories, to remember words," notes Patty Canac, who teaches olfactory aromatherapy at the Free School of Natural and Ethnomedicine (FLMNE), which I direct. Sometimes the restoration occurs in spectacular fashion. The therapeutic value of the work has been recognized, and similar work is now under way in a dozen medical centers as well as assisted living facilities for individuals suffering from Alzheimer's, Parkinson's, and multiple sclerosis.

Essential Oils in a Hospital Setting

The ability to use aromatherapy as treatment for Alzheimer's patients has been drawing the interest of a growing number of medical establishments. In France, hospitals in Colmar, Poitiers, and Valenciennes, as well mobile teams of palliative care companions in Rennes and Angers, and even retirement homes, have employed olfactory aromatherapy as a treatment support in cancer, geriatrics, and Alzheimer's. Benefits include the encouragement of sleep with lavender, soothing anxieties and agitation with petitgrain and orange zest, stimulating appetite with lemon, mood regulation with ylang-ylang and clary sage, increasing vitality with rosemary, and reducing nausea or pain with ginger and peppermint. The effect of essential oils for olfactory purposes, as shown in several studies, is quite concrete. Their influence can be felt on the autonomic nervous system, the central nervous system, and the endocrine system, and their effects are clearly visible on the patient's state.

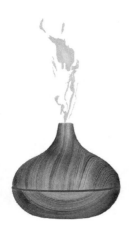

2

Cerebral Lesions and Their Consequences

A Look inside the Anomalies of the Alzheimer's Brain

ALOIS ALZHEIMER first described the illness that bears his name in 1906. At that time, knowledge of the brain and its diseases was not very far advanced, and Alzheimer's description of the condition does not correspond exactly to the disease as we know it today. Our understanding of brain function and disorders has evolved, and today we know Alzheimer's disease to be a neurodegenerative illness, an insidious and progressively evolving dementia with specific cerebral lesions: senile plaques and neurofibrillary tangles that disrupt the normal functioning of neurons and eventually lead to their death.

For a long time, the only sure method of diagnosing Alzheimer's with any certainty was when the patient's brain was on the anatomic pathologist's table. By autopsying the brain tissue, the pathologist could detect both the major alterations as well as the small signs specific to this disease. This is how Alois Alzheimer, when he examined the brain of a deceased patient, first identified the unusual characteristics (which were later recognized as typical of this disease) that gave birth to this new disease, or rather to the first elements of knowledge about it.

Over time, we have learned more and more about the cerebral lesions of Alzheimer's disease thanks to the modern techniques of medical imaging. We know, for example, that their development is gradual and generally progresses over a long period. Some neurologists break down their development into as many as eleven stages; clinical manifestations appear during the last three stages.

We also know that the lesions cause a growing cerebral atrophy that is spread out but predominant on the temporal lobes. The attack targets both the gray matter, which indicates the loss of neurons and dendrites, and the white matter, which corresponds to the axons. Cerebral activity is thus reduced, particularly in the temporal, prefrontal, and parietal regions.

The lesions caused by Alzheimer's do not affect all the regions of the brain in the same way. Their appearance and extension proceed in a predetermined manner. They almost always appear in the region of the hippocampus (so called because its shape resembles that of a seahorse), which plays an essential role in memory and emotional experience.

To better grasp the development of the disease and its symptoms, it is worth knowing where these lesions are located and how, little by little, they are able to take over the entire brain.

THE LIMBIC SYSTEM

The limbic system, which is attacked at the onset of Alzheimer's disease, is involved in both emotions and memory and therefore permits a link between memories and behavioral reactions. It receives and treats information by decoding it, comparing it, and adapting it to the situation.

This system is subdivided into numerous zones in different lobes of the brain. The limbic structures that are most involved in Alzheimer's disease are the hippocampus and amygdala.

The Hippocampus

The hippocampus gathers and processes information in connection with our verbal memory and visual memory. (Verbal memory understands the memories associated with what we have read, said, or heard; visual memory is used to recognize objects, faces, and places.) It is this zone of the hippocampus where Alzehimer's disease begins.

The hippocampus is thought to have developed among the earliest vertebrates some several hundred million years ago. It had an extremely important mission: the instant memorization of where to find food or where an enemy might be lying in wait and to record this memory in a durable fashion. An animal incapable of remembering this data died of starvation or was eaten by a predator!

Everything we perceive is stored in the hippocampus so that we can remember it beyond the time when we experienced it. The geographical and temporal memory capacity of the hippocampus lasts a lifetime. On the other hand, its ability to memorize content—in other words, what we have experienced or thought—is more temporary and generally restricted to around one day. Throughout our evolutionary history, the hippocampus never had any need for a greater memory capacity because we also have another storage space at our disposal: our long-term memory, which resides in the neocortex. Every new experience is first processed by the hippocampus and then transferred to long-term memory. This operation is performed during deep sleep. Our conscious mind must, in fact, be deactivated for this process to be successful. Otherwise, dreams and reality would become commingled, causing hallucinations or other unpleasant effects.

The Amygdala

The amygdala is a part of the brain that is involved in our emotions, emotional learning, and memory. This region is also adversely affected by the lesions caused by Alzheimer's disease.

MACROSCOPIC ANOMALIES

In someone suffering from Alzheimer's, the anatomic pathological exam reveals two major changes: senile plaques and neurofibrillary degeneration.

Senile Plaques

These lesions occur in the space between neurons. The core of the plaques consists of abnormal deposits of the beta-amyloid A4 protein, surrounded by neuronal extensions in a state of degeneration. Beta-amyloid proteins are not innately harmful, but they become so when they can no longer be eliminated properly. The amyloid deposits increase in size and spread and eventually begin to disrupt neuronal circuits. Then the first clinical signs of the disease become detectable in the patient.

Neurofibrillary Degeneration

Tau proteins (*tau* stands for "tubulin-associated unit") are normally present in the brain to protect neurons. In Alzheimer's disease, an abnormal process sets off an alteration of the tau protein structure through phosphorylation—that is, the proteins carry a phosphate group. The abnormal phosphorylated tau proteins eventually cluster together to form pathological filaments in the cytoplasm of nerve cells, causing degeneration of both the cellular bodies of the neurons (neurofibrillary degeneration, strictly speaking) and their extensions (neurofibrillary tangles). This leads to the gradual destruction of the neurons and their eventual death.

Connecting the Anomalies to Alzheimer's

A direct connection between the senile plaques and the neurofibrillary tangles is highly likely. It is hard to say which of the two proteins (tau or amyloid) is responsible for Alzheimer's disease. In fact, it would seem that perhaps both proteins, in abnormal presentations, could unleash the disease. They would be simultaneously responsible for the destruction of brain neurons and their connections (synapses), thus bringing about atrophy of the brain.

In other words, for Alzheimer's disease to develop, we would need to see the conjunction of the two phenomena:

+ Abnormal phosphorylation of the tau protein with aggregation in nerve cells
+ Accumulation of amyloid peptides throughout the brain

This process begins in the hippocampus, then gradually spreads throughout the entire cerebral cortex. The death of an increasing number of neurons gradually causes the appearance of the characteristic clinical symptoms: loss of memory, trouble speaking, and behavioral disorders.

OTHER FACTORS FOR CHANGES IN THE BRAIN

The Microbiota

A new connection between the brain and the intestines has recently been demonstrated: it is possible for gut microbiota to cause the appearance of amyloid proteins in the brain, a characteristic sign of Alzheimer's as well as Parkinson's.

The secretion of amyloid proteins by our intestinal flora would cause the appearance of the same kind of proteins in the brain. These abnormal proteins cluster like balls of yarn that fill the neurons and are passed on from neuron to neuron, and between different regions of the brain, and even between different organs. They most likely cause inflammation (a defense reaction of the body's immune system) and the death of cells.

Our intestines contain more than three pounds of bacteria. This community of microorganisms, or microbiota, helps the body with digestion, immune function, and other processes, including fighting inflammation. These bacteria are essential to our very survival. But since 2002, we have known that some of them produce amyloid proteins, which help their proliferation, adherence, and resistance. Those receiving the most study are the "curli" proteins, a type of amyloid fiber secreted by *Escherichia coli* bacteria. The work of S. G. Chen and his colleagues (2016), among others, has suggested that these bacterial amyloids found in the intestines can lead to the appearance and aggregation of amyloid proteins in other locations in the body, such as the neurons of the brain. The exact mechanism remains enigmatic, and research continues.

Mitochondrial Alterations

Alzheimer's disease can also be seen as a disease of protein metabolism, in which cellular processes appear to be halted, as if frozen, a synonym for the death of the neuron and its vital organs—namely:

- ✦ The cellular membrane, which is responsible for exchanges with the outside
- ✦ The mitochondria, the power plants of the cell

The mitochondria use oxygen to produce adenosine triphosphate (ATP), the principal molecule for storing energy in cells. Cells use ATP to ensure the maintenance of the body's major functions (digestion, breathing, transmission of nerve impulses, and so forth). This energy that is initially intended for cellular life is henceforth diverted. In the event of an illness caused by cellular congestion or clogging (where the body fails to adequately clear toxins or cellular debris), this energy intended to power cells is diverted for almost exclusive use by the immune system through the reactions of hypersensitivity and the mechanism of phosphorylation-dephosphorylation of enzymes.

However, there is always a downside. The mitochondria produce wastes by burning oxygen. These wastes are oxygen's free radicals. These aggressive molecules are normally neutralized by the body's antiradical system. But as we age, our defenses against free radicals weaken. The result is oxidative stress, whose primary target is the mitochondria, resulting in a reduction of energy output that cannot help but have adverse consequences on health.

In particular, free radicals can alter cell membrane permeability and damage mitochondrial DNA. In fact, as a team of Spanish researchers (Podlesniy et al. 2013) found, patients at risk of developing Alzheimer's disease show a reduction of mitochondrial DNA in their cerebrospinal fluid (CSF)—that is, the fluid in which the brain is immersed—at least ten years before the first signs of dementia appear. The reduction in mitochondrial DNA levels reflects the reduction of the mitochondria's ability to meet the energy needs of neurons, which alone consume 85 percent of the energy produced in the brain. Under these conditions, the neurons can only wither and die, one after another.

To function optimally, the mitochondria need nutrients that protect and support them. Antioxidants like alpha-lipoic acid, vitamins C and E, flavonoids, carotenoids, selenium, and glutathione protect against oxidative stress, while supportive nutrients like the B vitamins, L-carnitine, and magnesium have a positive effect on the energy output of mitochondria.

NB: it is believed that the mitochondrial genome is completely broken down after 125 years of life. This would therefore indicate the theoretic absolute limit of human longevity.

Phosphorus's Involvement

In Alzheimer's disease, tau proteins in the cytoskeleton contain an abnormal level of phosphorus (which is why they are called hyper-phosphorylated), and they aggregate to form thick filaments that hinder neuron function and eventually cause their death. Under normal conditions, phosphorylation is the biochemical mechanism put into play by the mitochondrial respiratory chain (also known as the electron transport chain) to synthesize proteins (enzymes, hormones, cytokines, genes) and, eventually, ATP. In Alzheimer's, however, we see that overactivation of that respiratory chain leads to hyperphosphorylation.

In part, this hyperphosphorylation arises from excessive antigen levels in the body. If Alzheimer's disease is caused or triggered by oxidative stress, as we have discussed, then it becomes possible to see that it is partially an iatrogenic disease (caused by antigens arising from medications) and partially a heteroimmune (or xenoimmune) disease (caused by exogenous antigens from the environment, arising from things like air pollution and food toxins). These antigens cause congestion of the body's cellular terrain. When the body is confronted by this chronic multitude of antigens, its demands on the immune system become a permanent phenomenon and we see a ramping-up of immune system activity. The body works to boost phagocytosis, which increases its oxygen consumption and thus its use of the mitochondrial respiratory chain. The respiratory chain requires phosphorylation; chronic excessive activation of the respiratory chain triggers hyperphosphorylation.

It should be noted that the list of neurotoxic environmental antigens grows longer every day with the constant arrival of synthetic products.

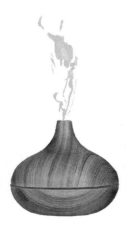

3

How to Establish the Diagnosis

A Multidisciplinary Approach

ALZHEIMER'S DISEASE is generally diagnosed in people starting at the age of sixty-five. Generally only half of people with Alzheimer's are ever diagnosed, and those who are not can find themselves lacking proper care for their condition.

The first signs of cognitive decline, though still imperceptible on a daily basis, appear around the age of forty-five. And forty-five years later, at the venerable age of ninety, one out of three people will have developed a senile dementia like Alzheimer's! The important point is therefore knowing how to take action on the trajectory of our cognitive aging process. The good news is that there is a long period of time during which we can eliminate or greatly delay the potential cerebral degeneration we fear threatens us.

DEFINING DEMENTIA

The term *dementia* has often been associated with madness or insanity, and for this reason it has taken on a pejorative connotation, with all the shame and rejection that entails. Today, generally speaking, we use the term *dementia* to mean a cerebral impairment whose symptoms are serious changes in the cognitive capability, emotional state, and social behavior of the patient. Dementia can be caused by chronic alcoholism (such as in Gayet-Wernicke syndrome), in which case cognitive capabilities can be restored through abstinence. It can also be due to severe cranial trauma after an accident, vascular problems after a stroke, Alzheimer's, and more. The causes for cognitive decline are legion and varied. Before starting treatment, getting a proper diagnosis is key.

Vascular Dementia

In industrialized countries, one-third of all cases of chronic dementia stem from a disturbance of the blood supply to the brain. The cause is usually damaged blood vessels, and for this reason this form of dementia is called vascular dementia. The damaged blood vessels leave the very sensitive neurons starved for oxygen, which leads to the destruction of a large quantity of nerve cells.

The vascular damage can be caused by a single serious episode, like a stroke, where a major blood vessel was obstructed. In the majority of cases, though, vascular dementia is the result of a long series of little strokes that go unnoticed until they have finally destroyed as much nerve tissue as a serious stroke. With any stroke, blood vessels shrink and harden, hindering blood flow. The resulting loss of nerve cells adversely affects cognitive function.

Alzheimer's Dementia

In other cases—which is to say, almost two-thirds of all patients—the chronic dementia is in fact Alzheimer's disease. Contrary to vascular dementia, which can appear and manifest anywhere in the brain, Alzheimer's begins in a clearly circumscribed region of the brain, the hippocampus, and then expands into other areas of the brain.

✧✧✧

Dementia, with its various clinical forms (including Alzheimer's disease), is inscribed in the great international classifications of mental diseases, including the fifth edition of the *Diagnostic and Statistical Manual of Mental Disorders* (a.k.a. the DSM-V), the bible published by the American Psychiatric Association. The diagnostic criteria described therein are those used by all the experts and researchers who specialize in Alzheimer's and similar diseases.

However, the term *dementia* is going to experience new evolutions. It is not applicable to what takes place during the first stages of the disease, and not all patients with Alzheimer's inevitably sink into a demented state.

MILD COGNITIVE IMPAIRMENT

Between normal function and the symptoms characteristic of the disease, an intermediate state has been identified that is not consistent with the diagnostic criteria for Alzheimer's. This state is characterized by a mild cognitive impairment and the onset of memory loss. Memory issues in the elderly are common, of course, but they are also often trivialized, even though they can be an early symptom of authentic memory disorders that correspond with the first stages of Alzheimer's (and other similar diseases).

In reality, the significance of mild cognitive impairment is controversial. For some, it corresponds to the predementia phase of Alzheimer's; 15 percent of subjects with mild cognitive impairment evolve toward a probable diagnosis of Alzheimer's. For others, though, it is merely a clinical syndrome whose causes and significance are variable.

Subjective Memory Complaints
Subjective memory complaints are self-reported problems with memory—momentary lapses or difficulties in recall—that can present

without any diagnosable cognitive dysfunction. Some people complain of not being able to find the right word in a conversation. Others complain of losing the thread of a conversation or not being able to remember a name: "I had it on the tip of my tongue." Others lose their keys, their glasses, their bills—or even the notebook where they write down what they don't want to forget.

Subjective memory complaints are a frequent phenomenon for senior citizens, but they are usually benign, meaning that they do not betray the presence of any cerebral affliction and don't represent a particular risk for Alzheimer's disease. It is normal to become forgetful. Life would be impossible if we had to remember all the information around us . . . and the capacity of our hard drive, large as it may be, would be quickly overwhelmed.

A defect in acquiring a memory may be connected to an absence of motivation (we don't retain what doesn't interest us) or a lack of attention (for example, when we are preoccupied or anxious).

Nevertheless, it is absolutely necessary to speak up about memory lapses. If these difficulties with memory mark the beginning of a cognitive disorder such as Alzheimer's, this early stage of development is the best time to start treatment. If they mark a hidden depression, it can be uncovered and treated properly.

Memory Complaints of Concern

One isolated lapse in memory has little value. A combination of problems should raise an alarm. They include:

+ Repeated loss of objects that a person set down a short time before
+ Difficulty keeping track of the time or day
+ Emotional disturbances

Another cause for concern is when people find that events of the recent past do not get recorded into memory, and they are not able to memorize new information. They may easily remember events that took place awhile ago, or even memories of the distant past, such as their childhood, but they are unable to recall what happened in the hours or days that have just passed.

Another symptom of alarm is a person who has memory issues but appears to have little concern about them, minimizing the consequences, blaming their age for their difficulty, and insisting that these issues have no bearing on everyday life and are not causing any problems.

THE MULTIDISCIPLINARY APPROACH

It is only possible to get a diagnosis of Alzheimer's by pursuing a multi-disciplinary approach. It should include a neuropsychological evaluation, brain imaging, a neurological exam, an overall medical assessment, a psychiatric exam if necessary, and a battery of clinical tests. The average period between the appearance of the first signs of trouble and the delivery of a diagnosis is about two years.

It was once standard to say that the Alzheimer's disease diagnosis was a diagnosis of elimination, since the medical profession did not have any single method of diagnosis at their disposal. Their approach was to exclude (and treat) all the ailments that cause memory impairments, and if that approach failed, after consultation with a memory specialist, the diagnosis could then be turned toward neurodegenerative diseases like Alzheimer's.

The approach remains the same for achieving a reliable diagnosis, but there are diagnostic criteria that the clinician will pull together over the course of a clinical and biological examination. Brain imaging scans are especially important (progress in brain imaging has made it possible to better grasp the connections between brain lesions and clinical disorders). They also make it possible to fine-tune an earlier diagnosis. Exploration of the various sectors of memory and other cognitive functions is also essential. A neurologist will then gather together the different clinical approaches and scans and refine the diagnosis.

It is difficult to identify the symptoms and then immediately link them to a diagnosis at the end of an initial assessment, especially in the early stages of the disease. The symptoms are essentially subjective. Even the neurological exam will yield normal results for a long time. It is only in advanced stages that obvious problems, like disorientation, abnormal movements, and difficulty walking, appear.

THE GENERAL PRACTITIONER'S EXAMINATION

A patient who is experiencing cognitive dysfunction that may be Alzheimer's, even if the symptoms are mild, should see their general practitioner for assessment. The most important purpose of the general practitioner's exam is to identify other potential causes for the cognitive issues so that they can be investigated. These include vascular issues, such as high blood pressure, high cholesterol, and diabetes; other physical ailments, such as anemia, a dysfunctional thyroid, infection (urinary, pulmonary), malnutrition, or heart disease; sensory deficits (sight, hearing); and certain pharmaceutical medications, such as proton pump inhibitors, bisphosphonates, statins, and alpha and beta blockers. All these disruptions of health can encourage mental confusion and disorientation, even without a direct link to Alzheimer's.

The exam begins with an advanced oral history, in which the physician digs into the patient's background to shed some light on the current situation. In the event that dementia is suspected, the physician may want to question people who are close to the patient, as the patient may not be able to remember exactly how their symptoms progressed or may not be aware of all the symptoms that have appeared.

The physician will order biological tests, starting with blood and urine, to track down pathological conditions that can cause cognitive disorders: vitamin deficiencies, hormone deficiencies (thyroid, adrenal gland), dehydration, anemia, diabetes, infection, or poisoning (heavy metals, food additives). Once identified, the bulk of these disorders are reversible when treated.

The findings from all these exams will make it possible to begin a diagnosis. In the event of doubtful or imprecise results, and all that remains is memory impairment, the exams can be performed again nine months later.

Making a diagnosis requires time that most general practitioners today don't have and procedures with which they are unfamiliar. If doctors are aware that the first sign of Alzheimer's disease is an olfactory disorder, this observation can help them gain valuable time for diagnosis and treatment. Otherwise, it will be a long hill to climb during which a succession of medical professionals will engage in establishing a diagnosis and starting a treatment. This path is very steep.

THE SPECIALISTS

The diagnosis of Alzheimer's disease is often random, especially at the beginning. While it can start with a general practitioner, it requires the services of a multidisciplinary team. To confirm the diagnosis, the patient will meet with various specialists, like a neurologist, psychologist, psychiatrist, geriatric medicine specialist, and speech therapist.

A patient who is suspected of having Alzheimer's will often be sent by their general practitioner to consult with a neurologist. The neurologist's initial assessment has several objectives:

✦ To specify the difficulties the patient is experiencing and their effect on the patient's mind, such as the presence of anxiety or depression

✦ To specify the nature and severity of the memory lapses and to identify whether the patient is having any difficulty with speaking (aphasia), performing gestures (apraxia), and object recognition (agnosia), which is most often determined by using standard cognitive screening tests (see below)

✦ To determine the stage of the disease

THE EXAMS USEFUL FOR MAKING A DIAGNOSIS

The indications for the use of these exams are based on the patient's symptoms. Not all of them are necessarily helpful. The two that are usually most helpful are the neurophysiological exam and brain imaging. The best diagnostic strategy combines the data gained from brain imaging and the neuropsychological evaluation with tests to determine the levels of Alzheimer's-specific biomarkers (total tau protein, phosphorylated tau protein, and beta-amyloid).

The Neuropsychological Exam

This assessment is performed by a neuropsychologist, usually in an appointment at a memory care center or hospital. It is essential for identifying the type and magnitude of impairment of the patient's cognitive functions. This term, *cognitive functions,* covers a long list of intellectual operations performed by the brain, including not only the various forms of memory (short term and long term) but also language, calculation, judgment, mental organization, orientation in space and time, and the perceptive functions (body image, spatial relations, recognition of objects and people, and so forth).

For Alzheimer's disease, diagnosis is based essentially on a series of three cognitive screening tests: the Mini-Mental State Examination (MMSE), the five-word test developed by B. Dubois et al. in France, and the clock drawing test. The tests are adapted to individual patients based on their sociocultural experience and the progression of the cognitive dysfunction. The earlier this evaluation is performed, the more specific it needs to be so as to reveal problems that might otherwise go unnoticed.

Mini-Mental State Examination (MMSE)

The MMSE is the most common cognitive screening test, and it is considered to be the standard clinical test used throughout the entire world. While it does not make it possible to make an etiological diagnosis, it does allow a comprehensive assessment of cognitive function and, together with the other assessments described in this chapter, can help clinicians diagnose dementia, evaluate its severity, and monitor its progression.

It consists of thirty questions that explore:

✦ Orientation in time and space
✦ Short-term memory
✦ Attention
✦ Ability to solve problems
✦ Speech (words, comprehension, reading, writing)
✦ Constructive praxis (execution of motor actions coordinated for a specific purpose)

The interviewer may ask, for example:

What is the year?
What is the season?
What is the month?
What is the date?
What day is it?

What hospital are we in?

What city/town are we in?

What country are we in?

What state are we in?

What floor are we on?

The interviewer will then ask the patient to perform simple tasks like recalling three words that were given earlier, counting backward from 100 by subtracting 7 each time, and identifying certain common objects.

Every correct answer counts for one point. The result is based on correct answers, with a top score of 30. A score below 24 is generally indicative of some form of dementia. But as noted above, the MMSE on its own does not diagnose dementia. Follow-up tests and further evaluations are needed for confirmation.

The Five-Word Test

The examiner says five words. The patient repeats them back to the examiner. If necessary, the examiner may give clues to help the patient memorize the words. This test explores only memory. It is simple and quick. The examiner evaluates how well the patient remembers the words over various lengths of time.

The Clock Drawing Test

This test calls for the examiner to give the patient a specific time, and the patient must draw a clock inside a pre-drawn circle to indicate that time (drawing the little hand and the big hand to indicate quarter after five, for example). This test explores several cognitive functions: semantic memory, executive function and praxis, spatial-temporal orientation, attention span, and visual-spatial awareness.

The examiner uses four criteria to evaluate a possible impairment of memory:

Is the number twelve at the top of the clock face?
Are twelve numbers depicted?
Are there two hands?
Was the time drawn correctly?

If one of these four criteria was not met, then a more extensive assessment will be necessary. This is a very sensitive but nonspecific test.

Neuroimaging

Today it is possible to directly see the different brain structures and their activity by means of various brain imaging techniques. In their materials on the early detection of Alzheimer's, the Alzheimer's Association breaks down the different forms of neuroimaging into three categories—structural, functional, and molecular—and describes them as follows:

Structural imaging provides information about the shape, location, and volume of brain tissue. Structural imaging techniques include computer tomography (CT) and magnetic resonance imaging (MRI).

Functional imaging reveals the extent to which cells in different regions of the brain are performing by assessing how well the cells use sugar (glucose) or oxygen. Functional techniques include positron emission tomography (PET) and functional MRI (fMRI).

Molecular imaging uses short-lived radioactive tracer compounds to detect cellular or chemical changes in the brain that are associated with various diseases. Molecular imaging technologies include PET, fMRI, and single photon emission computed tomography (SPECT).*

Some of these forms of neuroimaging are used rarely. We'll look at the more common ones here.

Magnetic Resonance Imaging (MRI)

This method gives much more precise results than computed tomography, especially for evaluating the onset of atrophy in the regions of the hippocampus and for detecting the accompanying vascular lesions, but it is more expensive and is contraindicated under some circumstances.

MRI is the preferred imaging examination for the etiological diagnosis of dementia. In Alzheimer's disease, it can show the existence of a cortical atrophy (and help discover atrophy in the hippocampus).

However, cortical or subcortical atrophy is not specific to Alzheimer's disease. MRI also makes it possible to rule out other causes, such as tumors, strokes, intracerebral or subdural hematomas, or ethylmalonic encephalopathy.

Computed Tomography (CT)

This method uses X-rays like ordinary radiography. It makes it possible to visualize brain structures through successive cross sections (tomography) on several different planes. It involves a simple examination centered on the hippocampus, the first region affected by Alzheimer's disease. It also makes it possible to eliminate certain diagnoses, such

---

*These are the imaging techniques known to be useful as of this book's publication date, but our technology, like our understanding of the disease, continues to evolve. See "Earlier Diagnosis," in the "Research and Progress" section of the Alzheimer's Association website, for a more in-depth discussion and updates.

as a brain tumor or stroke. It also provides morphological clues about neuron loss in areas that have become atrophied.

A CT scan is used when an MRI is contraindicated or not possible to carry out. It is not as precise as an MRI, but it makes it possible to rule out the other, curable causes cited above.

Positron Emission Tomography (PET)

PET scans offer a glimpse of the functional activity of various regions of the brain. This activity can be disrupted even before alterations to the brain structures are visible to a CT scan or MRI.

PET scans can be used for blood perfusion studies. In this evaluation, radioactive tracers are injected into the blood. The scan then measures the resulting radioactivity in the various regions of the brain, which tells us the blood perfusion (blood input) of each region. Neurons consume the glucose and oxygen that are supplied to them by the blood. Because they do not hold any reserves, the activity of a region can be seen immediately by the rate of its blood perfusion. In Alzheimer's disease, PET scans typically show a reduction of blood input in the hippocampus and neighboring posterior zones, meaning that these regions are less active.

Spinal Tap

A spinal tap is a method for taking a cerebrospinal fluid sample with a puncture of the lumbar region of the spinal cord. Analysis of the fluid can measure the concentration of three extremely reliable biomarkers for Alzheimer's: total tau (t-tau), phosphorylated tau (p-tau), and beta-amyloid 1–42.

Total tau: normal if below 450 pg/ml
Phosphorylated tau: normal if below 60 pg/ml
Beta-amyloid 1–42: normal if above 500 pg/ml

As reported by O. Hansson et al. (2006) in *Lancet Neurology,* "relative risk of progression to Alzheimer's disease was substantially increased" in patients with mild cognitive impairment and abnormal levels of these biomarkers in their cerebral spinal fluid (CSF). "The association between pathological CSF and progression to Alzheimer's disease was much stronger than, and independent of, established risk factors including age, sex, education, APOE [apolipoprotein E] genotype, and plasma homocysteine."

Electroencephalogram (EEG)

An EEG measures the electrical activity of the brain—that is, brain waves. It records the electrical activity of each brain region individually and in succession and presents this information as a series of wavelike patterns that can be read from left to right. Any alterations in the pattern, in comparison to another, makes it possible to identify a possible pathology on the corresponding cerebral zone. These anomalies can be alterations in the rhythm (faster or slower) or the amplitude (increased or reduced) of the recorded pattern.

In the case of Alzheimer's disease, the pattern is completely disrupted, with the EEG showing a general slowdown in the rhythm and an overall reduction in the amplitude on all the tracings, sometimes with more prominent changes in the posterior (occipital) region.

Even still, EEG anomalies that are indicative of Alzheimer's must be matched by brain imaging to confirm a diagnosis of Alzheimer's disease.

Fundus Examination: Retinal Imaging

We may soon be able to detect Alzheimer's disease in the depths of the eyes. The retinal and optic nerves are direct extensions of the brain and are connected to the occipital lobes. Many studies (see, for example, Campbell et al. 2017) have found that in Alzheimer's patients, beta-amyloid plaques appear not just in the brain but also in the retina, at levels proportional to the stage of the disease. Retinal analysis may make it possible to identify and map out the numerous (often in the hundreds), very small plaques and then to make a follow-up examination after treatment to see if the plaques have shrunk. Moreover, it may make it possible to see whether beta-amyloid is affecting the retinal vessels (and, by extension, the brain vessels)—an important point because, incidentally, when beta-amyloid is present in the blood vessels, it can, in rare cases, lead to hemorrhages.

GENETICS

Genetics does have an effect on our risk of contracting Alzheimer's disease, but our fate is not inevitably inscribed in our DNA. To evaluate a person's genetic risk for Alzheimer's, a genetic profile must be established. But first, it is necessary to make explicitly clear that carrying a "genetic risk" does not mean "hereditary." A genetic anomaly is not necessarily going to trigger the appearance of this disease in a person or their descendants. It most likely requires the combination of several factors, which are not all known.

Thanks to the ongoing scientific inventory of the human genome, it is now possible to isolate four genes that are involved in the genesis of this disease, while knowing that other genes are surely involved and will make it possible for us to better understand this disorder in the future.

The first gene to be identified is located on chromosome 21. A mutation here, in the coding gene for beta-amyloid protein, will cause it to be abnormally split and to establish itself in the amyloid plaques. These abnormalities are found in only 4 percent of the so-called familial forms of Alzheimer's, which are early onset.

There are also genes on chromosomes 14 and 1 that have been

linked to Alzheimer's. Like the gene on chromosome 21, these genes come into play in the early-onset familial forms of the disease, which are rare.

With respect to the more common and later-onset forms of Alzheimer's disease, an anomaly has been discovered on a fourth chromosome—chromosome 19. Here we find a gene that codes a protein known as apolipoprotein (APOE). APOE plays a role in the metabolism of lipids and the transport of cholesterol. It can be found in the general population in three forms consisting of two alleles. Alleles are copies of a gene. We inherit two alleles for each gene, one from our mother and the other from our father. These three forms are called APOE2, APOE3, and APOE4, which, by combining their alleles two by two, will appear in six possible combinations and six different genotypes. The most common form is APOE3. But it is APOE4 that is involved in the appearance of Alzheimer's disease.

APOE4 is an aggregation factor (of proteins) that over time encourages the formation of amyloid plaques. Being an APOE4 carrier constitutes a risk of developing the disease. Like all risk factors, its presence is not a guarantee of developing the disease. Carrying one copy of APOE4 (inherited from one parent) increases the risk of contracting Alzheimer's to 30 percent. Carrying two copies (inherited from both parents) raises this risk to 50 percent (and up to 90 percent, in some studies). These figures are to be compared to the only 9 percent chance of developing Alzheimer's among people who do not carry APOE4.

OLFACTORY TESTS

Olfactory impairment represents an early marker of this neurodegenerative disorder inasmuch as shortfalls, as made evident by the tests of detection, identification, discrimination, memory, and recognition, are observed during the first stages of the disease, before the appearance of other cognitive and behavioral symptoms.

As Liana Baltzer (2016) tells us:

> The precocity of olfactory impairment in Alzheimer's disease leads to the question of their presence in the presymptomatic form, and of their potential value as a predictive factor. A trial study carried out with 1,604 subjects, first-degree relatives of patients suffering from Alzheimer's disease and asymptomatic carriers of the E4 allele of the APOE4 gene, showed, after two years of observation, a significant correlation between the initially lesser olfactory capacities and the cognitive development of the disease. The risk of developing cognitive decline is in fact four to five times more likely among the subjects who presented with a reduction of olfactory capabilities than among the normosmic subjects. This suggests that an olfactory test could be one of the alternatives to more expensive methods (CT scan, etc.) for early diagnosis of Alzheimer's disease.

Olfactory Testing with Essential Oils

In aromatherapy, an individual's uniquely personal sense of smell is the standard reference for identifying which essential oils will work best for that person. We can take advantage of that singular response to test and monitor the olfactory capacity of someone whom we suspect may be in the very early stages of Alzheimer's disease.

To begin, select a maximum of three essential oils that the person is able to identify and recognize. It is best if the scent is somehow connected to the person's life experience—if it is a "scent memory" that calls forth an emotional response. Absolutes can also be used, as they are also effective in olfactory therapy. Avoid all synthetic scents.

To present the essential oil to the patient, place a drop on a smelling strip and have the person sniff it. Ask the person to identify the scent and recall its connection to their life experience. Repeat the test, over time, and monitor the results.

The Olfactory Stress Test

Peter Schofield and his colleagues in Newcastle, Australia, have suggested that an olfactory "stress test" could detect presymptomatic Alzheimer's. They administered atropine, an anticholinergic, into the nasal passages of test subjects and found that it caused a more substantial reduction in olfactory performance in subjects with known or suspected Alzheimer's than in those who were not experiencing any dementia symptoms. They theorized that this sort of olfactory stress test, which is simple and inexpensive, could make it possible to detect this disease.

Could we use the sense of smell as a diagnostic tool to facilitate treatment of Alzheimer's at an early stage? Such an approach could have tremendous benefit for the patient. We know that 95 percent of Alzheimer's patients have impaired olfactory function, and this consistent, widespread sign could put us on the road to early diagnosis and treatment. Perhaps it is the missing link that makes it possible to explain the origins of the disease.

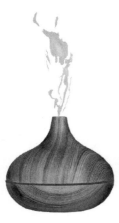

4

Laboratory Analysis

Biochemical Factors for Diagnosis, Prevention, and Treatment

LABORATORY ANALYSIS of blood samples can detect various causes for memory disorders and thus identify ways of treating them. In fact, several diseases that can cause memory impairment can improve if the source at fault is treated.

Though these pathological conditions are involved in only 1.5 percent of all cases of cognitive issues, no one can solve a problem whose nature remains a mystery. If we wish to prevent Alzheimer's disease, it is imperative that we identify all of its possible signals so that we can take steps that will lead to the best possible outcome.

Laboratory analyses of patients presenting with cognitive symptoms, like memory loss, show less-than-optimal values for a large number of factors related to brain function. A person enjoying good health can have three to five markers that show signs of impairment. But that number is generally much higher in people who present with cognitive disorders. In this chapter, we'll look at those markers and their possible connection to Alzheimer's.

HOMOCYSTEINE

Homocysteine is a common amino acid that is formed from the breakdown of protein. It is found in fruits with hulls, lamb, beef, cheese, turkey, pork, fish, crustaceans, soy, eggs, green beans, and dairy products.

Normally, homocysteine is converted in the body into methionine or cysteine (other amino acids). This recombination requires vitamin B_{12}, vitamin B_6, folates, and betaine. When the body's stock of these B vitamins and betaine is low, homocysteine collects in the body and damages blood vessels and the brain. Homocysteine is neurotoxic, especially for the hippocampus, and especially when stimulated by glutamate. Elevated homocysteine is a known risk factor for heart attack, cerebral atrophy, and Alzheimer's disease.

Homocysteine levels higher than 6 micromoles per liter (μmol/1) can present a risk, and the higher the level, the greater the risk. These elevated rates eventually will cause cognitive decline and atrophy of the hippocampus. On the other hand, homocysteine levels can be modulated with exercise and supplementation with B vitamins.

VITAMIN D

Vitamin D is a fat-soluble vitamin that is synthesized in the body by the skin through the effect of ultraviolet radiation on cholesterol. Though estimates vary, researchers agree that vitamin D deficiency is a global problem. In the United States alone, more than 40 percent of the population is deficient in vitamin D. A deficiency in this vitamin would be a factor in the development of neurodegenerative disorders like Alzheimer's disease and Parkinson's, as well as osteoporosis, depression, and cancer.

Ideal blood levels of vitamin D (measured in the form of

25-hydroxycholecalciferol) fall in the range of 20 to 40 nanograms per milliliter (ng/ml). Low levels can be corrected by supplementation with a plant-based form of vitamin D₃. Take it with fatty food to support its metabolism. Also take advantage of the beneficial effects of sunlight for natural vitamin D production, such as by enjoying outdoor activities, like gardening, during the day.

TRACE ELEMENTS

Zinc

Zinc is a trace element that is essential for our body because it is involved, directly or indirectly, in all metabolic processes.

A zinc deficiency is a triggering factor for Alzheimer's, taking into account the many biological functions of this trace element. For example, it blocks excessive release of glutamate and thereby protects the neurons of the hippocampus. Furthermore, a deficiency in zinc will hinder neurogenesis in the hippocampus.

A rise in zinc levels goes hand in hand with a reduction in levels of copper, which is suspected of being a factor in Alzheimer's disease or accelerating its development. For this reason, if you're having zinc levels analyzed, it is also a good idea to have the concentration of free copper analyzed. Customarily, we require a copper:zinc ratio that is less than 1:2. In addition, because iron is a powerful inhibitor of zinc's absorption into the body, iron and zinc should never be combined in the same multivitamin complex.

Selenium

Current methods of agricultural production inhibit the presence of selenium; therefore, selenium deficiencies are far from scarce. However, this metalloid plays a major role in the fight against free radicals. It comes into play as a support for the immune system, and it has a chelating effect against toxins and heavy metals like mercury, lead, arsenic, silver, and cadmium. In combination with essential fatty acids and vitamin E, it plays a role in anti-inflammatory and blood-thinning actions. Through its many actions, and especially its antioxidant properties, selenium makes it possible to fight against the processes of cerebral aging.

In Alzheimer's patients, selenium levels can be 50 percent less than in normal subjects. The best food sources for selenium are Brazil nuts, whole grains, garlic, onions, leguminous plants, egg yolks, and brewer's yeast, but selenium must be administered in much higher than nutritional doses to produce therapeutic effects. Researchers suggest a daily oral therapeutic dose of 200 μg, which is four times higher than the daily recommended intake for adults (50 μg). The two forms available are chelated selenium (selenomethionine) and selenium yeast (yeast enriched with selenium).

Lithium

By activating neurogenesis in the hippocampus, lithium acts as an antidepressant. Furthermore, it fights excessive secretion (and thus the aggregation) of beta-amyloid.

We should note that bipolar disorder—for which lithium is often prescribed—is associated with an increased risk of Alzheimer's.

Our foods contain very little lithium. Lithium can be useful in the event of an anxiety attack. Here in France, I recommend the product Granions de Lithium.

INFLAMMATION MARKERS

Sedimentation Rate

The sedimentation rate is the rate at which erythrocytes (red blood cells) settle out, or become sediment, in a sample of blood as a measure of inflammation. Inflammation causes cells to clump, which means they settle faster, so an increased sedimentation rate indicates inflammation in the body. It is a common, proven, simple test. All illnesses cause inflammation in the body and therefore an increased sedimentation rate. The normal range is generally 0 to 22 mm/hour for men and 0 to 29 mm/hour for women, with age and pregnancy being factors that lean toward the upper end of the spectrum.

C-Reactive Protein (CRP)

CRP is a protein manufactured by the liver. Its synthesis increases substantially in the event of any inflammation in the body's cellular terrain. So, like the sedimentation rate, CRP levels can be used as a gauge of inflammation in the body. Normal levels fall under 12 mg/L.

The high-sensitivity C-reactive protein (hs-CRP) test is the best option for anyone suffering from dementia-like issues. This test can detect much lower levels of CRP and serves as a gauge of chronic inflammation, rather than inflammation related to a specific trauma or infection. CRP levels as measured by a hs-CRP test should be lower than 1 mg/L. If it is higher than this, the source of the inflammation must be determined. It might be, for example, a cardiovascular problem, a diet with excessive sugar or bad fats (trans fats), intestinal hyperpermeability (leaky gut), gluten sensitivity, or some specific toxins. Once the source has been identified, the inflammation should be neutralized and then another hs-CRP test performed.

Cytokines

Cytokines are inflammation mediators, and high levels of cytokines in the blood indicate inflammation somewhere in the body. To illustrate their importance, I have chosen to describe three of them: IL-1, IL-6, and TNF.

Interleukin-1 (IL-1)

IL-1 is the central mediator of both inflammation and immunity. It is produced by the immune cells (B and T lymphocytes, phagocytes, neutrophils and eosinophils, monocytes, and macrophages).

Interleukin-6 (IL-6)

IL-6 induces the production (by the hepatic cells) of the proteins of the acute phase of inflammation, such as, for example, C-reactive protein, whose serum rate correlates, incidentally, to that of IL-6. The primary characteristic of IL-6 is activation of the vascular endothelium by increasing its procoagulant properties, which brings to mind the vascular lesions and coagulation anomalies observed in hyperhomocysteinemia.

Tumor Necrosis Factors (TNF)

TNF (alpha and beta) is involved, like the other cytokines, in the mechanisms of autoimmune diseases.

Omega-3 and Omega-6 Essential Fatty Acids (EFAs)

TNF and IL-1 secretions are regulated by the polyunsaturated fatty acids of the omega-3 type, whose importance in the regulation of inflammation and immune processes is no secret. This observation confirms, once again, if there is any need, the role of good nutrition in maintaining good health.

We must also examine the omega-6 and omega-3 ratio in red blood cells. Both fatty acids are important for health, but omega-6 EFAs encourage inflammation (they are pro-inflammatory) and the omega-3s are anti-inflammatory. The omega-6:omega-3 ratio should be lower than 3:1 but not lower than 0.5:1, as this would increase the risk of hemorrhage.

HORMONE STATUS

Thyroid Hormones

We frequently encounter thyroid disorders in Alzheimer's disease. When thyroid function diminishes, the body produces more thyroid-stimulating hormone (TSH) to cause the thyroid to produce more hormones. This is why elevated TSH can be an indication of an under-active thyroid (hypothyroidism).

The normal range for TSH is somewhere between 0.4 and 4.2 mIU/L (that's milli-international units per liter). Levels higher than 5 mIU/L are evidence of hypothyroidism, in which case all metabolic processes are slowed. When TSH falls below 0.01 mIU/L, this is evidence of hyperthyroidism: metabolism is accelerated, hence the necessity to rein in the gland.

Free T3 (triiodothyronine) is the active thyroid hormone, but its life span is short; its molecules will disappear within a day's time. Optimal levels for this hormone are between 3.2 and 4.2 pg/ml (picograms per milliliter).

Free T4 (thyroxine) is essentially the form of the thyroid hormone when it is stored in the body (for the purposes of metabolism, the body transforms it into T3). Its life span is around one week. The optimal range falls between 1.3 and 1.7 ng/dl (nanograms per deciliter).

Levothyroxine is sometimes prescribed for hypothyroidism, but I do not recommend it. It provides only a synthetic T4 hormone, which rarely converts to the active T3. Thyregul (my exclusive formula, available in France) is much preferable. It contains six cofactors that transform T4 into active T3.

Estrogen and Progesterone

The role of the different forms of estrogen (estradiol, estriol, and estrone) and progesterone in cognitive function is sometimes controversial, yet their effect is quite striking!

Estrogen, in particular, is a key factor in the prevention of dementia. A deficiency of this hormone doubles the risk of developing Alzheimer's disease. And when the ratio of estradiol and progesterone is elevated, it can cause cognitive problems.

Ideal levels are as follow:

Estradiol: 50–250 µg/ml
Progesterone: 1–20 µg/ml
Estradiol:progesterone ratio: 1:10

THE BIOLOGICAL EFFECTS OF STRESS

Stress is inevitable in daily life. It can offer us a boost in times of duress, but when it becomes chronic, it is one of the primary factors of cognitive decline.

A stressful event causes the release of the stress hormone adrenaline. But when stress becomes chronic, adrenaline gives way to another hormone, cortisol, which, in excess, disrupts proper brain functioning.

Pregnenolone

Pregnenolone, produced by the adrenal glands, is considered the main steroid hormone in the body. It is the starting material for the sexual steroids, like estradiol and testosterone, and for the stress hormones, like cortisol and DHEA. During periods of heightened stress, the body focuses its use of pregnenolone to produce stress hormones, which prevents the production of sex hormones at optimal levels.

Pregnenolone protects the neurons. Low levels of this hormone are a risk factor for cognitive decline.

Cortisol

An elevated cortisol level—a stress response—forces the body into action, with negative consequences for the brain and memory. To begin, it interferes with the metabolism of carbohydrates (sugars), which are the essential nutrients for neurons (energy). It also allows calcium to penetrate cells, which leads to calcification and disrupts neuron activity. Calcium's penetration causes magnesium to leak out of the cells, and it is then eliminated by the kidneys. This can cause a serious magnesium deficiency.

In this way, elevated cortisol levels damage neurons, which makes chronic stress an important factor in hippocampus deterioration and, consequently, cognitive decline.

DHEA

DHEA is considered a "neurosteroid" that becomes mobilized during times of stress. It is generally measured in the form of DHEA sulfate. Concentrations of this hormone decrease steadily with age, reaching its lowest levels around the same age that neurodegenerative disorders often present.

Cortisol, pregnenolone, and DHEA sulfate can be measured easily in blood serum, saliva, or urine collected over a twenty-four-hour period. Optimal levels are as follows:

Morning cortisol: 10–18 µg/dl
Pregnenolone: 50–100 µg/dl
DHEA sulfate: 350–430 µg/dl for a woman,
    400–500 µg/dl for a man

NEUROMETABOLISM: BIOMARKERS

As described in chapter 3, cerebrospinal fluid (CSF) can be tested for beta-amyloid and tau protein levels, which are biomarkers for Alzheimer's. Normal levels are generally considred to be:

Beta-amyloid 1–42: 500–1500 pg/ml
Total tau protein: 100–450 pg/ml
Phosphorylated tau protein: lower than 60 pg/ml

HOW TO DETECT A NEUROLOGICAL OR PSYCHIATRIC DISEASE

We have three tests available to us for depression and a number of psychiatric and behavioral disorders, including not only Alzheimer's disease but also bipolar disorder, autism, hyperactivity, schizophrenia, and more.

Histamine

Histamine is a neuroregulator that ensures negative feedback on the release of neurotransmitters in the synapses. The amount of histamine in the blood makes it possible to identify a methylation problem. In fact, histamine is converted into methylhistamine by physiological processes.

In the case of hypomethylation, the level of histamine in the blood remains elevated. When hypermethylation is the problem, the histamine level is reduced.

The optimal histamine values are between 400 and 800 ng/L. When histamine levels are elevated (histadelia), the release of neurotransmitters is arrested and their rate diminished. When it is low (histapenia), the release of neurotransmitters is elevated and their levels increased.

Hypomethylation is essentially corrected by increased intake of s-adenosyl-L-methionine (SAM-e), a universal methyl donor.

Hypermethylation is primarily corrected by increased intake of B group vitamins (B_3, B_6, B_9, and B_{12}), which activate demethylation enzymes.

The Copper:Zinc Ratio

As discussed earlier in this chapter, the copper:zinc (Cu:Zn) ratio must be less than 1:2.

As both copper and zinc are essential for health, it is important to study them together. The zinc ion is full of electrons, whereas the copper ion does not have enough. Consequently, copper transports electrons into the many proteins that contain it and generates a source of free radicals that cause damage to the membranes.

Zinc, which is present in more than three hundred different proteins, does not produce free radicals.

Kryptopyrrole

The standard values are usually below 200 µg/L.

Kryptopyrroles are metabolites resulting from an abnormality in the synthesis of heme, a precursor to hemoglobin whether of genetic origin or acquired. These pyrroles bind with zinc and the active form of vitamin B_6 (pyridoxyl-5-phosphate, or P5P), which causes a reduction of these nutrients that are essential for the synthesis of neurotransmitters.

The deficits can be corrected by supplementation with vitamin B_6 and zinc, which will cause a drop of kryptopyrroles levels and help improve the symptoms caused by the deficiency.

Correction of such biochemical anomalies must be adapted to individual requirements. The optimum doses can vary between individuals.

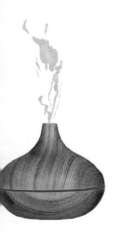

5

The Brain and Its Neurons

A Primer

HOW MANY MYTHS, mysteries, and fantasies have been spun about the brain, which governs our every thought and gesture! It contains:

+ The central nervous system, consisting of the encephalon housed in the cranium and its extension, the spinal cord, which descends along the backbone
+ The peripheral nervous system, consisting of the cranial nerves connected to the encephalon and the spinal nerves connected to the spinal cord
+ The autonomic nervous system, which controls automatic (unconscious) physiological functions and contains two components that perform opposing activities, the sympathetic and parasympathetic systems

Seen from a distance, however, the nervous system functions are quite simple. They follow this schema: Bits of sensorial information, known as afferents, arising from both the outside environment and the internal milieu, arrive at an integration center—that is, the central nervous system. This system processes the information and then sends out a motor response, known as an efferent. Information, integration, and response bring cellular networks into play; they communicate with one another through electrical and chemical signals.

THE DEVELOPMENT
OF THE BRAIN

The human brain has been subject to profound changes taking place over millions of years.

The Reptilian Brain

This is our most archaic brain, where the life instinct and the programming of the species are located. This is the headquarters for all the innate behaviors that ensure survival. It has no conscience and feels no emotion. This is the stage where snakes, turtles, and so forth have remained.

The Limbic Brain

According to the systematization of the archencephalon, this aspect of the brain is formed by a grouping of very deep nervous centers at the center of the encephalon. They are closely linked, but this brain also contains the associative cortical zones, the thalamus, the hypothalamus, and the prefrontal regions.

Functionally speaking, the territories of the limbic brain are responsible for the organization of fundamental instinctive behaviors and the expression of emotions and motivations ensuring the protection of the individual and the survival of the species. This is the domain of instinct.

In short, it performs three primordial functions:

+ Living (dietary motivations)
+ Surviving (fight or flight response and the protection and preservation instinct)
+ Reproduction (sexuality)

According to the study of phylogenesis, the limbic brain corresponds to the combination of the archencephalon and the paleoencephalon. It thereby forms the rhinencephalon (olfactory brain) of the macrosmatic mammals—those with an excellent sense of smell, for whom this sense is an essential function. The olfactory function in human beings is reduced, but all the other functions of the limbic lobe have been preserved.

The limbic system includes the following organs:

+ Olfactory bulbs: Neural structures located in the forebrain. They receive neural input from the cells in our nasal cavity and pass it along to the brain.
+ Hippocampus: Essential to memory and emotional experience. (See chapter 2 for more details.)
+ Amygdaloid complex: A cluster of nuclei located in the anterior part of the temporal lobe and involved in emotions, emotional learning, and memory.

Both the hippocampus and the amygdaloid complex are stricken by the lesions caused by Alzheimer's disease.

THE STRUCTURE OF THE BRAIN

From a structural perspective, the brain, or encephalon, consists of the outer meninges (membranes), the brain itself, and the cerebral ventricles, which are filled with cerebrospinal fluid. In the brain, we find two types of matter:

- ✦ Gray matter, which consists of the neuronal cell bodies and axons (extensions) and is located to the outside or periphery of the brain
- ✦ White matter, which consists of nerve fibers (some wrapped in myelin sheathing) and is located beneath the gray matter

The Cerebral Hemispheres

The left and right hemispheres make up the upper portion of the brain and represent more than 80 percent of its mass. The two hemispheres are separated by a longitudinal fissure in which the falx cerebri is folded, but they are joined at the lower end of this fissure by a large connecting "cable," the corpus callosum.

Though the two hemispheres appear to be similar anatomically, they are quite different on the functional plane, with a clear distinction between the right brain and the left brain. The left hemisphere receives sensations and governs the motor function of the right side of the body, and vice versa. Right-handed people are said to have a dominant left hemisphere, and vice versa.

Five Lobes per Hemisphere

Seen from outside, the cortex resembles a walnut half, with relief areas, or cerebral convolutions (gyri) separated by grooves (fissures) that vary in depth. These convolutions permit the cortex a surface area of around six and a half square feet (whereas it would be less than five square feet if the cortex were smooth, like that of a rat).

The cortex is divided into two hemispheres, which are connected by neuron extensions that ensure their integrated function and form the corpus callosum. Deep furrows divide each hempisphere into five lobes, each of which is named after the bone of the cranial cavity over it. To

illustrate this division and naming of the lobes, let's look at the temporal lobe, under the temporal bone at the side of the skull; the parietal
lobe, under the parietal bone at the roof of the skull; and the frontal
lobe, under the frontal bone that forms the forehead.

The Temporal Lobe

This lateral region of the cerebral cortex receives auditory information
and manages things learned recently—that is, our immediate memory.
It is connected to the limbic system. Impairment of the temporal lobe
causes short-term memory problems and makes it difficult for us to
recall recent events. In addition, we can become lost in a familiar environment. We may suffer from a reduced vocabulary and have trouble
finding the right word. Later, we may have hesitancy in recognizing
known faces, objects, and places.

The Parietal Lobe

This region is located in the upper median part of the cerebral cortex
and is involved in several different functions of the brain: treatment of
spatial information, our sense of direction, information related to body
image, and the consistent organization of actions.

The Frontal Lobe

The frontal lobe, found in the anterior region of the cerebral cortex,
is involved in planning and in forms of higher thought. It allows us
to take initiative and to plan and organize our actions. It also controls
our social behavior and values. Impairment here will interfere with our
sense of judgment.

The Cerebral Cortex

This part of the brain, the "orchestra conductor" of the nervous system,
joins together all the so-called higher cerebral functions:

+ Initiation and control of intentional movements
+ Sensory perceptions: touch, pain, temperature, hearing, sight, taste, smell
+ Mental activities: memorization, speech, understanding and learning, reasoning, thought, and so forth

The cerebral cortex consists of five types of functional zones:

+ The sensitive zones, which receive and decode all the sensory messages from the periphery
+ The olfactory zone, which receives the flow of information about odors arriving from the nasal cavities, through the olfactory nerve (the first cranial nerve)
+ The zone of taste, which receives the flow of information from receptors located on the upper surface of the tongue
+ The motor zone, which directs intentional movements
+ The associative zone, where complex mental activities originate

NEURONS

Neurons are the primary constituent elements of the brain. The rest of the brain consists of glial cells (astrocytes, oligodendrocytes, microglia, ependymal cells, Schwann cells, and so on), which are support cells responsible for feeding and protecting the neurons. There are around thirty billion neurons in our brain and around twice as many glial cells.

A neuron consists of several parts:

+ A cellular body, consisting of cytoplasm (surrounded by a cellular membrane) and a nucleus, which contains DNA
+ Dendrites, formed from branches extruding from the cellular body and connecting with many other neurons

✦ An axon, or nerve fiber, a long extension of the cellular body that can reach a dozen or more inches in length

Neuronal Signal Transmissions

A neuronal axon carries a nerve impulse—an electrical charge—away from the cellular body and transmits it to a neighboring neuron through the intermediary of a synapse. The electrical signal, upon reaching the synapse, triggers the release of a neurotransmitter into the intersynaptic space. This neurotransmitter travels to a neighboring neuron, where it triggers the production of a nerve impulse, which in turn flows along that neuron's axon until it reaches the following synapse, and so on.

This "electrical current" permits the brain to coordinate movements, control breathing, and express hunger, pain, joy, or sorrow . . . provided that it is able to flow. Anything that interferes with the free flow of nerve impulses impedes cognitive function.

Brain activity begins with a stimulus: a thought or a piece of information arriving by way of one of the five senses. When this stimulus reaches the brain, the brain sends messages to the rest of the body via the spinal cord and nervous system. Each component plays a specific role, but it is always the electrical current that is the vector for the information being transmitted.

Thousands of dendrites connect neurons to one another, thereby forming the body's electrical network. Although the neurons are very close to one another, they do not touch. The tiny space that separates them is called the synaptic cleft. The junction between two neurons is a synapse. We each possess more than one hundred billion synapses. The axon of a neuron carries the chemical mediators, or neurotransmitters, that cross through the synapses in order to reach the dendrites of the following neuron. It is this movement, or flow, that allows electrical current to pass from neuron to neuron.

Neurotransmitters attach themselves to neurons through specific receptors. We can compare the receptors to a lock-and-key mechanism: each receptor "lock" is receptive to only one neurotransmitter "key." A neurotransmitter locking into a receptor is a specific communication. These chemical mediators therefore ensure the delivery of the electrical signals that transmit information to the rest of the body.

Neuron Capital

We are born with a set amount of neurons—our "neuron capital"—and that number shrinks through the normal aging process of the human being. However, contrary to what was once believed, it has been shown that some neurons are able to develop out of stem cells even after birth; this process is known as neurogenesis. This phenomenon concerns certain cerebral regions like the hippocampus.

We shall discuss neurogenesis at greater length in chapter 11, where we address the brain's plasticity.

NEUROTRANSMITTERS

The brain and the rest of the organism function most optimally when each neuron is correctly programmed to produce, send, and receive specific chemical mediators. The four chemical mediators that are essential to our physical and mental balance are:

+ Dopamine
+ Acetylcholine
+ Gamma aminobutyric amino acid (GABA)
+ Serotonin

Together, these and other neurotransmitters form the code of our brain. Each one creates unique electrical patterns that can be visualized in the form of brain waves. The study of these waves and their interrelations provides the data necessary to explain a variety of physiological and encephalic symptoms. It is then possible to detect a dysfunction by a specific biochemical imbalance.

Acetylcholine and serotonin seem to be the two neurotransmitters that are the most seriously disrupted in Alzheimer's disease. The disease is characterized by a reduction in acetylcholine levels as well as an anomaly affecting certain cellular receptors of acetylcholine (called nicotinic receptors). This reduction is caused by an enzyme, acetylcholinesterase (AChE), which breaks down or hydrolyzes acetylcholine.

Serotonin levels are also often reduced in Alzheimer's patients. Serotonin is the hormone that promotes calm and tranquillity. It helps us manage stress, our emotions, and our balance, and it also helps us curb our impulses and regulates appetite and sleep. It makes it possible to keep our impatience and irritability in check.

To have a sufficient quantity of these neurotransmitters, it is necessary to add the following to the diet:

1. Precursors—the amino acids the body uses to make these hormones. For acetylcholine, that's choline, phosphatidylcholine, or phosphatidylserine, which are primarily found in soy lecithin. For serotonin, it's tryptophan or 5-hydroxytryptophan (5-HTP), which can be found in small quantities in fish, grains, cauliflower, pineapple, bananas, broccoli, spinach, walnuts, soy, carrots, chocolate, and mung beans.
2. The good fats, meaning omega-3 and omega-6 fatty acids as well as phospholipids. They allow for good synthesis of the precursors as well as providing good membrane fluidity, which allows the precursors to leave the synapse.
3. Probiotics, to ensure good intestinal microbiota and digestion.
4. Co-factors: magnesium, zinc, copper, and vitamins B_6 and C.

5. Antioxidants, which protect the cellular membrane receptors that will receive the neurotransmitters.

All of these elements need to be taken into consideration when Alzheimer's disease is involved, because all the neurotransmitters are important for good brain function.

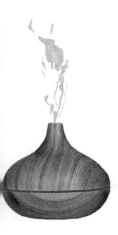

6

A Stroll Down Memory Lane

The Systems and Stages of Memory

BRAIN DISTURBANCE due to disease can be revealed through three types of syndromes: cognitive disorders (intellectual), character and behavioral changes, and their effects on daily life.

Cognitive functions are those that allow us to understand and take action in the world: memory, speech, execution of gestures, recognition of objects and people, and the ability to comprehend abstraction, to plan, to monitor tasks and their goals (executive functions), and so forth. Cognitive functions make it possible for us to harmoniously integrate into the outside world, with those around us, our surroundings, and our milieu.

One particular cognitive function is central: memory, whose role is to acquire, store, and utilize the different pieces of information that we collect. While it is true that all the cognitive functions rely on each other, it is especially true that memory is central to our experience with and our ability to function in the world. Disorders of memory, such as Alzheimer's disease, have a powerful effect on our cognitive function as a whole because all other cognitive functions rely on it, to varying degrees.

THE FIVE SYSTEMS OF MEMORY

Memory is based on five systems:

+ Perceptive or sensory memory
+ Working or short-term memory
+ Semantic long-term memory
+ Episodic long-term memory
+ Procedural memory

Though different, these types of memory and the neural networks that govern them are interconnected and rely on each other. This complex unit, as a whole, is essential for identity, expression, knowledge, learning, reflection, and even individual projection into the future.

Perceptive Memory

Perceptive memory in human beings depends on sensory modalities, especially sight. We are scarcely aware of this memory system's functioning. It makes it possible for us to retain the knowledge of sounds and images, without even realizing it. This is the memory that allows us to return home out of habit thanks to visual references. It allows us to remember faces, voices, places, and smells.

Our extremely sensitive and effective sensory receptors (visual, auditory, olfactory, gustatory, and tactile) all capture information from the outside world and transmit this information toward specific zones of the brain. The transmitted information is then given a quick analysis. This operation is essential when we think of the profusion of information we experience from the outside world in every moment of the day. Unfortunately, this sensory memory lasts for only a handful of milliseconds—or, for visual perception, somewhere on the order of 200 milliseconds.

Brief as it is, sensory memory is then passed on to our working memory, better known as short-term memory.

Working or Short-Term Memory

Our working memory makes it possible to retain information for the time necessary to use it (for example, remembering a telephone number long enough to dial it or holding a sentence or paragraph in mind long enough to understand it). Working memory is, in fact, the memory of the present. It allows the retention of information for several seconds to dozens of seconds. Demand is put upon it constantly.

In most cases, the neurobiological mechanisms connected to working memory will not permit long-term storage for this kind of information; memory of them is quickly forgotten. Nevertheless, there are interactions that take place between the working memory system and our long-term memory. They permit memorization of certain events and thereby allow us to recall memories when confronted by certain similar situations so that we can better adapt our response to them.

Working memory is indispensable in daily life. Though it is a far cry from the extreme brevity of perceptive memory, working memory can hold information for twenty to thirty seconds. Once it has been dealt with by the working memory system, information that is deemed worthy of storage is passed along to our long-term memory system.

Long-Term Memory:
Semantic and Episodic Systems

Long-term memory makes it possible for us to acquire basic knowledge about ourself (our history and personality) and the world (geography, politics, current events, nature, social relations, and even professional experience). This is the memory of learning and knowledge. It concerns the personal data that is accessible to our consciousness and can be expressed. This set of memories spreads across a long span of life. This system's purpose is to create engrams of information in such a way so that it remains available when we want it.

What we see, hear, feel, smell, and taste will be recoded in a definitive manner in this long-term memory. But the implementation of this memory system depends on the starting point of the recording process. There are two options: semantic memory and episodic memory.

If the starting point consists of cultural or general knowledge, we store that information in our semantic memory, a form of long-term memory that corresponds to general concepts and knowledge that are unrelated to our personal experience but still necessary for us to remember.

If the starting point consists of dated and localized memories that correspond to specific episodes from our own life, we store that information in our episodic memory. This system makes it possible to recall past moments (autobiographical events) and to foresee the days ahead. In fact, whether we ask a person to bring up a memory that took place several months ago or to think of their upcoming vacation and imagine what is going to happen then, the same cerebral circuits are activated.

Scent memory—having an aroma bring up a particularly sharp remembrance of an event associated with it—is a form of episodic memory. We see it in the Proust phenomenon, a sudden, involuntary autobiographical memory triggered by a scent and named for the author whose work provides a fine illustration of the importance of smell in autobiographical memory, with the idea that scent is the last rampart of memory.

The details of episodic memories get lost over time. The features that are common across different life experiences become amalgamated into knowledge that is no longer connected to a particular event. The bulk of episodic memories therefore transform in time into general knowledge.

These two forms of permanent memories—semantic and episodic—are categorized as declarative and explicit. In effect, we can draw them from stored memories with conscious intention. When we question these memories, we can verbalize the answer.

Procedural Memory

Procedural memory holds our knowledge of activities that we do automatically. It is what allows us to drive, walk, ride a bike, or ski without having to relearn the skill every time. Artists and athletes rely on this system of memory to perfect their processes and achieve excellence. These processes are performed implicitly, or unconsciously. We cannot really explain how we proceed, how we maintain balance as we ski downhill without falling. The movements are made without any conscious control; the neural circuits are on automatic.

NEURAL NETWORK FUNCTIONING

From the neurological point of view, there is no one single memory center in the brain. The different memory systems bring distinct neural networks into play. These networks are observable by medical imaging when involved in the tasks of memorization or the recovery of memories.

These networks are interconnected, nonetheless, and function in close collaboration. The same event can have both semantic and episodic content, for example, and the same piece of information can be represented explicitly or implicitly.

MAKING A MEMORY

Several stages mark the journey of information from experience to memory: encoding, storage, consolidation, and restoration.

Encoding

All new information enters the brain through the intervention of the sensory organs. It is treated, coded, and transformed into a mnemic trace potentially suitable for storage. The first stage, encoding, places particular demand on the left frontal lobe. The effectiveness of the encoding process depends on how alert we are and on our motivation and emotional state.

According to the most widespread theories at present, encoding entails translating the information that is connected with our activities and motivations into the language of the nervous system. Among these bits of information, there are some that are of value for only a short time and erased quite quickly. This short-term memory is quite limited temporally (ranging from several dozen seconds to a couple of minutes) as well as in content (it is measured by our ability to repeat it immediately—for example, a series of numbers in the order in which they were given).

Storage

Once it has been encoded, the information is sorted. Bits that we don't need to remember are erased quite quickly. The rest—the memories we want to retain—is stored. This operation takes place in the neocortex and will be effective only if the consolidation stage functions correctly.

The storage processes seem to be hard to observe through brain imaging because they involve these consolidation mechanisms. Nevertheless, the hippocampus seems to play a central role in temporary storage and in the longer-lasting storing of explicit information.

Memorization is the result of an alteration in the connections between the neurons of a memory system. That capacity for alteration is known as synaptic plasticity. When a piece of information reaches a neuron, proteins are produced and carried toward the synapses to reinforce them and create new ones. This produces a specific network of neurons associated with the memory that is engraved into the cortex. Each memory therefore corresponds to a unique configuration of the spatiotemporal activity of interconnected neurons. The representations are eventually divided within the vast, complex networks of neurons.

Regular and repeated activation of these networks allows these connections to be reinforced or reduced, with the consequence of either consolidating the memory or forgetting it. It is important to make clear here that forgetting is part of proper memory function, outside those cases involving disease.

As we age, the plasticity of the synapses becomes reduced and the changes of the connections become more ephemeral, which could provide an explanation for the growing difficulties we have in retaining information.

Consolidation

The hippocampus comes onto the stage to ensure successful consolidation. It serves as a crossroads, or zone of transit, that organizes the information of the brain and makes a definitive copy from what was a temporary copy. It forms part of a neural circuit whose role is to distribute the information related to the memory in the neocortex, where it is stored once and for all. It is a veritable transformer/adapter of the information in memory.

The hippocampus's capacity for geographical and temporal memory lasts a lifetime. On the other hand, its capacity to memorize content—what we experienced or think—is limited temporarily to a few hours. Our new experiences arrive in the hippocampus and then are transferred to long-term memory. This operation takes place during deep sleep. In fact, our consciousness needs to be deactivated for the process to be successful, so that dreams and reality do not become commingled.

Restoration

The term *restoration* refers to the recall of a memory. When a memory emerges automatically, this operation is relying on the hippocampus. When the recuperation requires mental effort, it places its demand on the right frontal cortex.

The stored information can be restored in the form of memories or behaviors. The trigger for restoration may be internal clues, or free recall (I hear a song that seems familiar to me, and I try to remember the singer's name), or external clues (for example, being in the presence of a friend reminds me of a time when we had dinner together). The trigger may also be the re-presentation of information, or recognition (someone mention's a colleague's name, and I remember them).

For memory to perform well, all the component elements of the memory must be reassembled like a jigsaw puzzle. This is why all the aspects of making a memory—storage, coding, consolidation, and the structure and organization of all the components—are important. The better these subprocesses work, the easier it will be to pull together all the different elements to restore a memory in its greatest possible entirety.

WHEN THE TRANSFORMATION HAS FAILED

If the cells of the hippocampus or the pyramidal cells have been damaged or destroyed, the processes of transformation and restoration will not take place: the information is lost. This is what happens in Alzheimer's disease, in which the neurodegenerative processes damage the cells of the hippocampus and make all attempts at learning and memorization futile.

The memory disorders that are characteristic of Alzheimer's disease are connected to a deficiency in the processing of new information into episodic memory, whereas semantic and procedural memories will be preserved for quite a long while.

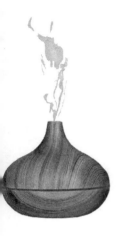

7

Development of the Disease

The Stages and Progression of Alzheimer's

WHILE THE PROGRESSION of Alzheimer's disease is unavoidable, the pace is variable depending on the patients and their individual circumstances, and it's generally slow.

It is customary to distinguish three stages of the disease, depending on the severity of the dementia: mild, moderate, and severe. Some neurologists divide out a fourth and final terminal stage, in which only palliative care is possible. But the definition of these stages is fairly vague and varies depending on whether the severity of the cognitive shortcomings and their ramifications in daily life are taken into account.

We know that the onset of the disease takes place ten to twenty years before any clinical signs appear, and we believe it initiates at about the age of sixty-five in 95 percent of cases. These are sporadic forms of the disease—which is to say, that other immediate family members are not touched by it. The remaining 5 percent of cases correspond to a familial form of Alzheimer's and start much earlier, well before the age of sixty-five.

Note: When memory disturbances are involved, it is essential to make a distinction between what is normal and what is caused by the onset of Alzheimer's disease. As discussed in chapter 3, mild cognitive impairment (MCI) is common in older people, and though such impairment may raise fear of Alzheimer's, it does not reveal the presence of a cerebral disturbance and does not systematically represent any particular risk of developing Alzheimer's disease.

COGNITIVE DEFICITS ARE THE HEART OF THE DISEASE

There is a large international consensus for defining the severity of the disease by using the Mini-Mental State Examination (MMSE), the standard test for quickly detecting cognitive deficits. The stages defined by this scale are only a gauge, but they are useful for categorizing the different stages of Alzheimer's disease.

As discussed in chapter 3, the MMSE has a top score of 30 points, with one point for every correct answer. The more points a person gets, the less likely it is that they have a cognitive deficit. A score of 25 to 28 points should raise suspicions of mild cognitive impairment. The red line is placed at 24 points; if the final score falls below 24, we must suspect a cognitive disorder compatible with a dementia syndrome and suggest a follow-up examination with a specialist.

A score between 20 and 24 indicates mild dementia, a score between 10 and 20 moderate dementia, and a score below 10 severe dementia. However, it is imperative to underscore the fact that a low score has no diagnostic value; it simply provides evidence of a reduction in cognitive performance and is no way specific to Alzheimer's disease. Furthermore, the score doesn't always reflect the severity of the cognitive shortcomings, which may be masked by other factors such as trouble with speech.

The cerebral lesions of Alzheimer's disease, like those of all neurodegenerative diseases, develop insidiously and very gradually. The definition of the stages is an approximation of the variability of the disease, depending on the patients and the evaluation criteria used.

THE PRECLINICAL OR MILD STAGE

The preclinical, or mild, phase is indicated when the MMSE score is higher than 20.

As the disease begins to take root, cerebral lesions form quite slowly, without causing any clinical symptoms. This preclinical phase is completely silent. It is estimated to last from fifteen to twenty years, or even more. Only the most sophisticated methods of medical imaging (such as PET scans) make it possible to identify two occurrences that are observable very early in the brain: a defect in the elimination of the beta-amyloid protein, which collects and becomes a neurotoxin, and a drop in the consumption of glucose in some cerebral regions, in particular those connected with memory and cognition (such as the hippocampus and amygdala).

The first symptoms are often confused with the normal effects of aging, but extensive neuropsychological tests can reveal mild cognitive impairment at least eight years before an individual starts exhibiting the diagnostic criteria of Alzheimer's disease. The complex activities of daily life are the first to be affected, accompanied by changes in behavior.

How do we know if a memory lapse is simply a common problem related to aging or stress or a sign of the onset of Alzheimer's disease? Most of the time, the little memory lapses we encounter are side effects of fatigue or stress. We find ourselves always doing one thing while thinking of something else, or multitasking, or rushing about. This causes cerebral exhaustion.

However, we should never neglect these little memory lapses, especially if they are persistent. If they persist even when fatigue or stress is no longer a factor, these memory disorders could be the consequence of physiological disorders, such as the beginning of the degeneration of the brain.

In the earliest stages of Alzheimer's, the memory lapses will be tied to recent occurrences, while older memories will remain perfectly intact. Patients may forget a rendezvous, someone they met, a film they saw the evening before, the shopping list, the burner left on under the saucepan, or a phone call they had to make. Additionally, they will exhibit an inability to learn and retain new information. Patients often minimize these issues or even hide them from their loved ones. Eventually, though, the symptoms become clear even to outsiders.

THE PREDEMENTIA OR MODERATE STAGE

The predementia, or moderate, phase is indicated when the MMSE score falls between 10 and 20.

When the cerebral lesions reach a certain stage of intensity and have extended their influence, other symptoms appear. By virtue of the lesions' initial assault on the regions of the hippocampus, we see not only memory lapses but also changes in behavior. Little by little these problems escalate, and other intellectual shortcomings may appear. Speaking and comprehension become slower, but day-to-day activities are normal, and only the most complex activities are affected. This predementia stage lasts for two to four years on average.

Memory's Twilight

The difficulty patients are having with memory becomes more and more obvious. They forget where they put things—their wallet, phone, keys, and other important objects. Explicit memory is attacked early, making learning a chore. More precisely, episodic memory is the most adversely affected, long before semantic memory, making it difficult for patients to retain memories of events from their life, especially those that happened recently.

Difficulties with Speech and Comprehension

Aphasia is the impairment of our ability to comprehend or use words, and about 40 percent of Alzheimer's patients experience it in this second phase. They may first have trouble with specific words, and then with sentences. They become incapable of expressing themselves correctly. They may say one word while meaning another, and their sentences become riddled with provisional words while they struggle to find the right ones. If they are aware of this problem, they may become annoyed and flustered and perhaps end up depressed and withdrawn.

These language problems can be summarized as an impoverishment of vocabulary and fluency. At this stage, patients are still able to communicate but only with more childish forms of expression. Writing becomes disrupted before speech. Patients will begin to make spelling mistakes, use only capital letters when writing, or jumble lowercase and uppercase letters. Their writing may become entirely phonetic, such as "nite" for "night." They may have trouble writing in a straight line. Later, they begin to have trouble reading. Eventually, they will not be able to write out or even sign a check.

Difficulties with comprehension compound the difficulties of communication. In the beginning, patients may ask for more elaborate sentences to be repeated, as if they had not heard them properly. Next, the meaning of words may escape them. People will feel obliged to repeat words and sentences for them, but in vain. Patients may blame their difficulty on hearing loss, which, incidentally, is common among those elderly people in whom these same problems with writing can be found.

Difficulties with Orientation

Orientation in time becomes impaired. Patients no longer know the day's date, the day of the week, the year, or the current season. Eventually, they may confuse day and night.

Orientation to place and surroundings also becomes a challenge. In a new location, patients find it harder and harder to get their bearings. When confronted by new situations, they find it hard to adjust. To avoid the danger and discomfort this disorientation raises for them, patients may be hesitant to leave familiar surroundings—their home or their neighborhood, for example. The disorientation worsens as the disease progresses. Eventually, patients may get lost even in their own homes.

Running Away

Almost 50 percent of Alzheimer's patients run away from home. This behavior is not simply a loss of direction but an intentional flight. To some extent, it corresponds to a quest to solve an inner sense of being ill at ease that arises from the combination of several cognitive deficits. However, thanks to their disorientation to time and place, and with the addition of panic, patients are not able to find their way home.

These runaway episodes have consequences that can be life-threatening. Preventive measures include securing the premises (locking doors and hiding the keys), having telephone numbers (for the police, hospitals, friends and family who can help with the search) handy in case of a runaway, and even the installation of a surveillance or security system.

Psychotic Disturbances

It is not rare for patients to experience hallucinations and delusional ideas during the course of this disease. Psychiatrists call these phenomena psychotic disorders.

Hallucinations

Some 20 percent of Alzheimer's patients experience hallucinations, customarily during more advanced stages of the disease. A hallucination is a perception of a phenomenon that exists only in the patient's mind. It is an "objectless perception." It is not the misinterpretation of a real object, like a painting in the living room that we think is alive or a floor lamp that we mistake for a person. Nor is it an "impression of a presence," when we feel there is someone in the room whom we cannot see.

Hallucinations occur when the brain is no longer able to decode the messages that the eyes project into it, and the unidentified images can destabilize the person. In Alzheimer's, the hallucinations are often visual. They can be elaborate, such as visions of people, animals, or complex scenes, or just fleeting sensations (a brief impression that a shadow or animal has popped up in the room). Patients may also experience auditory hallucinations and, more rarely, olfactory hallucinations (odors) and, even more rarely, tactile ones (the sensation of being touched).

Though hallucinations may seem terrifying to the people in a patient's life, such as when a patient sees, quite realistically, a person who is absent or deceased, people with Alzheimer's see them as normal and usually are not disturbed by them. These hallucinations are evidence that patients are no longer making any distinction between imagination and reality. They are living a kind of dream.

Delusional Ideas

Delusions are false beliefs that are held with absolute conviction but don't stand up to the test of reality. They can be seen in 20 percent of Alzheimer's patients, most often when the disease has progressed quite far. Normally they arise from feelings of jealousy ("I know that when you go out, it is to see your boy/girl friend"), abandonment

("You want to get rid of me"), or theft ("Someone has been in my apartment, and some things are missing"). These ideas can be quite perturbing when they are aimed at you or someone close ("I don't want to see my daughter anymore because each time she comes, she steals my little spoons or jewelry").

The term *delirious conviction* is used in these cases, based on a patient's certainty about everything they suggest, argue, and demonstrate. Attempts to reason with them obviously run smack into their absence of reason. In fact, families can make the situation worse by getting involved in a debate and trying to demonstrate through reason that the patient's beliefs are absurd, or, to the contrary, they can make the situation better by simply going along with what the patient is saying.

This is one of the greatest hardships of caregivers. They are conscious of the madness but are unable to accept that the people they loved or love are indeed crazy.

Motor Behavior Disturbances

Agitation

This term refers to forms of hyperactive behavior that can vary in their expression and meaning. Agitation is a symptom that can, in fact, betray mental disturbances or a physical malaise. It can be seen as the physical expression of anxiety, of a discomfort that the patient cannot express in words.

Agitation can be a significant problem in certain stages of the disease. Physical constraint and the administration of medications against a patient's will can be imposed as a last resort to spare the patient and the patient's caregivers.

It can require sustained observation to determine the true cause of a patient's agitation. Note that a fever, which can be one of the effects caused by the disease when inflammation is an issue, can trigger agitation.

The Initial Stages of Wandering

Wandering is the consequence of a patient's feverish need to walk. Walking behaviors, which are sometimes permanent, occur frequently but do not constitute any kind of problem as long as they are beneficial and allow the patient to maintain physical autonomy and get a change of scenery.

Some wandering states are a consequence of the prolonged use of neuroleptic medications that then generate contradictory reactions. Sleep becomes increasingly disturbed. The drugs that are provided to induce sleep or reduce the patient's agitation only aggravate the desynchronization of sleep.

THE DEMENTIA OR SEVERE STAGE

The dementia, or severe, phase is indicated when the MMSE score falls below 10.

When a patient's cognitive deficits start having a visible effect on everyday life, such that they require help with all of their daily activities, even the most ordinary ones, then the third stage, the so-called dementia phase, has been reached.

In accordance with the international definition, it is only when this stage has been established that a diagnosis can be made with sufficient probability (the clinical phrase is "probable Alzheimer's disease").

Patients at this stage often require placement in an institution because of their dependency, inability to communicate, and geriatric complications. Their cognitive functions have now vanished almost completely. They may lose the ability to understand or use speech. They often simply repeat sentences without understanding the meaning of the words. They are now incapable of forming any judgments or solving the most basic problems.

Depression

Depression in Alzheimer's patients can take several forms. Melancholy remains the most common, with its accompanying tears, self-deprecation, and pessimistic remarks. Apathy is also common. Another form, called active depression, which is especially common in male patients, manifests as an aggressive attitude; it may arise from patients feeling like they are drowning in anxiety, and so they lash out at the world around them.

While depression is frequent in the earlier stages of the disease, especially among patients who are aware of their growing deficits, it blurs once their intellectual functions decline past a certain threshold.

Higher Intellectual Abilities Are Stricken

Patients' faculties—their ability to form judgments, abstractions, mental calculations—become severely altered. They have trouble performing the activities of daily life. They begin displaying coordination problems with their limbs, especially in activities requiring the use of both hands. They can no longer use a corkscrew, hit a nail with a hammer, turn on the television or radio, get dressed, and so on.

Balance problems appear. Falls become frequent and pose a risk of broken bones.

Eventually, patients reach a stage of constant decline. They become completely disorganized, and severe mental confusion with hallucinations and delusions becomes commonplace. Also evident are appetite disorders, incontinence, and infections worsened by confusion, disorientation, and the use of sedatives.

Patients can now have episodes of violent behavior. A simple remark can trigger an ill-tempered reaction, but it can also be met with violent anger and uncustomary insults. Physical violence is rare, but it can occur when caregivers try to make a patient do something they don't want to do (such as use the bathroom) or prevent them from doing what they want, such as going outside.

Incontinence

This symptom appears quite late in the progression. It is necessary to identify any potential physiological causes, especially a prostate infection in a male patient. Neuroleptics can cause urine retention and, subsequently, overflow incontinence (when the bladder is full, it seeks to empty itself by forcing the sphincter open) in patients. The belly above the pubic region should be felt carefully for a "bladder globe," which would be the sign of a blockage.

Incontinence can also simply be the consequence of late-stage Alzheimer's. In this case, the patient has come to a regressive phase. Now, maintaining proper hygiene can be challenging, and the care required may seem overly intimate to the patient, and therefore aggressive or humiliating.

THE FINAL STAGE

In this stage, the terminal phase, Alzheimer's patients become entirely dependent on their caregivers. Evaluation of their cognitive function with the MMSE is no longer possible. Speech is reduced to a few simple sentences or words, which ends with a complete inability to speak. A certain amount of aggression may still be present, but most often patients suffer from apathy or fatigue.

Muscle mass and mobility decline to such an extent that patients are no longer capable of performing the smallest motor task without help. When the progression of the disease is not interrupted by a heart attack, stroke, or cancer, the deterioration becomes profound. Patients' language gradually becomes unintelligible, with constant moans and endlessly repeated gestures. They can no longer stand up or sit and become completely bedridden. They no longer recognize anyone. They need to be fed by hand. Incontinence is total. Patients often lie in a fetal pose, with eyes vacant, and are unable to swallow even liquid; wasting away in a state of cachexia heralds that their end is near.

After a time that can vary in duration, death ensues, sometimes by means of pneumonia, sometimes by choking when swallowing something down the wrong pipe, and sometimes by infection, such as a urinary tract infection or bedsores.

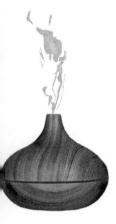

8

The Multiple Causes of Alzheimer's Disease

Medications, Mitochondria, and More

THE POTENTIAL CAUSES of Alzheimer's disease are, at this time, multiple, chiefly because it is still impossible to say for sure just what the causes are. As a baseline, evidence has been presented that some elements encourage the appearance of the disease. These elements are called risk factors, which means their presence provides a favorable environment for the disease to occur, but they are not determinative factors.

While the presence of a risk factor increases the possibility of developing the disease, it is crucial to realize that risk is only a statistic. A person can have one or more risk factors and never develop the disease, just as, vice versa, someone can develop the disease while not having any of the known risk factors.

ALZHEIMER'S AS AN IATROGENIC DISEASE

A host of epidemiological studies have shown a significant correlation between the consumption of certain synthetic medications and Alzheimer's disease. A team of researchers from France and Canada, for example, found a link between Alzheimer's and benzodiazepines. As they comment, "The stronger association observed for long term exposures reinforces the suspicion of a possible direct association, even if benzodiazepine use might also be an early marker of a condition associated with an increased risk of dementia. Unwarranted long term use of these drugs should be considered as a public health concern" (Billioti de Gage et al. 2014).

That is alarming, from the perspective of public health. Who among us isn't close to someone who relies on—or relied on—benzodiazepine antidepressants or sleeping pills? Many of them have become household names: Valium, Mogadon, Temesta, Lexomil, and others.

This is why the pharmaceutical industry has pulled back from sustained research on the brain: it is too complex. The vast domain of toxicology—especially pertaining to environmental and occupational forms—as well as the collection of unwanted effects of synthetic medicines when taken over long spans of time give us spontaneous experimental models for all the diseases caused by cellular clogging, especially the neurodegenerative diseases.

All chemical medications taken over the long term are not recognized by the body but instead are seen as invasive elements. They can cause leaky gut syndrome and oxidative stress through the production of free radicals. Oxidative stress is a perverse effect of the elimination mechanism and the phagocytosis of organisms that are foreign to the body. It is the price we pay for detoxification. It is also a potential factor in our risk for Alzheimer's, as we will discuss in a moment.

A variety of synthetic medications have been identified as possible culprits in Alzheimer's disease. They include:

All calcium channel blockers
Beta-blockers
Neuroleptics

Imipramine antidepressants

Statins (lipid-lowering drugs)

PPIs (proton pump inhibitors)

The majority of anticoagulants

Diuretics

Biphosphonates

Food additives and colorings identifiable by the letter E followed by a number

Medications for Alzheimer's Treatment?

Ironically, donepezil, the medication given to Alzheimer's patients under the trade name Aricept, works via an anticholinesterasic mechanism, meaning that it blocks the anticholinesterase enzyme, thereby preventing the destruction of acetylcholine after the passage of a nerve impulse. In effect, it prevents the neural receptor from detaching from the acetylcholine molecule to prepare for reception of a new acetylcholine molecule. The result is an accumulation of acetylcholine in the synaptic cleft and an interruption to the transmission of nerve impulses. This causes numerous signs of hyperstimulation of the nerve fiber through untimely depolarization of the postsynaptic membrane. The cholinergic receptor that is constantly meeting the demands of this parasympathetic chemical mediator eventually becomes detached from it.

Using chemical medications to treat Alzheimer's symptoms delays the completion of a true treatment for the cause and ends up inducing a phenomenon of therapeutic polypharmacy: the prescription of still more antigenic and aggressive medications that only cause the oxidative stress to worsen and overwhelm the immune system.

MITOCHONDRIA
AND ALZHEIMER'S DISEASE

As discussed in chapter 2, among patients with a risk of developing Alzheimer's disease, a reduction of mitochondrial DNA in their cerebrospinal fluid can be observed at least ten years before the first signs of dementia appear (Podlesniy et al. 2013). The reduction of mitochondrial DNA levels in the cerebrospinal fluid reflects the reduction of the ability of the mitochondria to fulfill the energy needs of the neurons, with subsequent loss of neurons.

Several factors may contribute to mitochondrial dysfunction. Primary among them are certain diseases and disorders, pathogens and toxins, and oxidative stress.

Diseases Connected to
Mitochondrial Dysfunction

Mitochondrial dysfunction is associated with all of the following:

Disorders on the autism spectrum
Bipolar disorders
Major depression
Schizophrenia
Migraine
Parkinson's disease
Multiple sclerosis
Cancer
Type 2 diabetes
Metabolic syndrome
Steatosis not caused by alcohol
Heart failure
Chronic fatigue syndrome

Fibromyalgia

Sarcopenia

Sleep apnea

In the end, this list represents a large range of afflictions that clearly affect more people than those with only genetic mitochondrial diseases. Any of them may be a contributing factor in the development of Alzheimer's disease.

Pathogens and Toxins

There are several categories of pathogens and toxins that are enemies of mitochondria:

* The modern diet, which encourages the consumption of excessive sugar, especially in the form of fructose, and not enough antioxidants (fresh fruits, dried fruits, oleaginous fruits, vegetables, spices, herbs, green tea)
* Xenobiotics—namely, pesticides, heavy metals, nanoparticles, medications (antibiotics, statins, acetaminophens, NSAIDs, vaccines)
* Germs, with honorable mention going to herpesvirus, the mitochndiral DNA killer (we'll talk more about it later in this chapter)

Oxidative Stress

The energy production process inside the mitochondria generates free radical wastes. These aggressive molecules are normally neutralized by a healthy internal defense system. With aging, this defense system toils harder and harder to hold back the proliferation of free radicals. The result is a state of oxidative stress whose main target is the mitochondria. Free radicals will gradually wear away the constituent parts of mitochondria, particularly its very fragile DNA. This causes a reduction in its energy production that will inevitably cause the loss of neurons and create problems with an individual's health.

THE APOE4 GENE

As described in chapter 3, there is considerable evidence for genetic factors that increase susceptibility to Alzheimer's disease. This is not to say that Alzheimer's is a hereditary condition predetermined by our genetic makeup but rather that certain mutations in genes can predispose us to the likelihood of developing the disease, though not necessarily causing it. People who carry these genetic risk factors may never develop the disease.

Specifically, the coding gene for the lipoprotein APOE, which is found inside senile plaques along with the beta-amyloid peptide and other proteins, has been identified as a genetic risk factor. A lipoprotein is a protein that carries lipids to the various nerve cells, which use the lipids to repair themselves. Research shows that the presence of the APOE4 form of this lipoprotein gives an elevated risk of Alzheimer's, and a concomitant risk for earlier development of the disease. The risk of developing Alzheimer's carried by APOE4 may be exacerbated by an unhealthy diet and lifestyle. From this perspective, the APOE4 genetic mutation could be looked at as something that accelerates the development of a disease that was triggered by an unhealthy lifestyle.

TYPE 3 DIABETES

PET scans show that in people afflicted by Alzheimer's, the metabolism of glucose in the brain is abnormal. It is slower than it is in individuals who do not have this disease. This same kind of abnormality can be seen in people who are genetically predisposed to diabetes even before they have exhibited clinical signs of this disease.

High rates of insulin and glucose are risk factors for developing Alzheimer's, in which a reduction of glucose consumption is clearly visible, especially in the frontal cortex and temporal lobes. And people affected by type 2 diabetes have a 50 percent higher risk of developing Alzheimer's disease in comparison to nondiabetics.

Insulin, a hormone released by the pancreas, regulates blood sugar levels. Cells normally, when under the influence of insulin, use the glucose that is present as a source of energy and store the excess in the form of glycogen. In type 2 diabetes, the cells are no longer able to do this despite the presence of insulin. They become insulin-resistant, and blood sugar levels increase in the bloodstream, although the pancreas continues to produce more insulin, but in vain.

In the mid-2000s, researcher and physician Suzanne de la Monte saw that brain cells in Alzheimer's patients displayed a loss of sensitivity to insulin that grew worse as their dementia became more severe. The neuron cells had become resistant to insulin, which explains why they were no longer utilizing glucose properly. She advanced the hypothesis that Alzheimer's disease could be a form of brain diabetes, which she referred to as "type 3 diabetes" (de la Monte and Wands 2008).

One Solution: The Ketogenic Diet

While glucose metabolism in neurons is impaired in Alzheimer's disease, an alternative fuel is available: ketonic compounds (or ketones), which the body produces by the breakdown of fats in the liver.

In fact, research shows that ketones may reduce the presence of beta-amyloid plaques and their neurotoxicity (Broom et al. 2019). And a ketogenic diet has been shown to improve both mitochondrial function and cognitive performance in elderly patients with Alzheimer's (Rusek et al. 2019).

Ketone bodies, produced mainly by the liver from dietary fat, include acetone, which is exhaled, and acetoacetic acid and beta-hydroxybutyric acid, which the blood transports to the different organs. Ketones are able to cross the blood-brain barrier and enter the brain, where they can be used as fuel.

Medium-chain triglycerides have the singular feature of producing more ketone bodies than long-chain triglycerides, and these triglycerides are absorbed more efficiently and transported directly into the liver. So enriching your diet with medium-chain triglycerides offers an enormous advantage: you can obtain the same amount of ketones as you would with the classic ketogenic diet, but by eating much less fat.

Medium-chain triglycerides (MCT) occur naturally in butter (which is about 9 percent MCT), goat's milk, and especially coconut oil, which, at about 60 percent MCT, has the highest triglyceride content of any food.

There are several more-flexible ketogenic diets available that are easier to follow over the long term by offering a wider variety of foods. They include the modified Atkins diet and the glycemic index diet.

Other Avenues to Pursue

Trials are under way with inhaled insulin, which would make it possible to increase brain insulin levels without changing the insulin content in the body. The results so far are encouraging.

We still need to learn why insulin is no longer operating properly in the brain in Alzheimer's patients. This could open new fields for investigation and prevention of the disease.

THE PATHOGENIC TRACK

Several studies have identified different infectious agents as possible risk factors for developing Alzheimer's disease. They include the virus that causes herpes type 1, the picornavirus, and bacteria like *Helicobacter pylori* (responsible for stomach ulcers), *Borrelia burgdorferi* (the bacteria responsible for Lyme disease), and *Chlamydia pneumoniae*. Fungal infections are also often found in the brains of Alzheimer's patients.

Normally, the brain is protected from pathogens circulating in the body by the blood-brain barrier, but this filter can weaken, especially in the case of chronic inflammation. Some germs can also gain access to the brain by way of the nose, the intestines, and even the eyes. In fact, Alzheimer's disease can be seen as a reflection of the brain's protective reaction to infectious or toxic attacks. Whether it arises from infection, toxins, or the accumulation of beta-amyloid and tau proteins, neuroinflammation (by which I mean all immune system reactions in the brain) triggers cognitive decline.

INFLAMMATION

While inflammation is a helpful immune reaction, one that is essential for the body's ability to stop the development of illness and eliminate foreign substances, the same cannot be said about chronic or persistent inflammation, which can degenerate into a disease. Obesity, cardiovascular diseases, neurodegenerative diseases, and often cancer display an inflamed cellular terrain over long spans of time (from several months to several years).

Chronic inflammation is often the consequence of the presence of aggressive elements like pesticides (from environmental and food exposure) and free radicals (from poor dietary habits).

The protective role of nonsteroidal anti-inflammatories against chronic inflammation and its long-term effects has been especially demonstrated in epidemiological studies of populations showing rheumatism-like pathologies. Patients who were treated by rheumatologists and had taken a lot of nonsteroidal anti-inflammatory drugs (NSAIDs) showed a reduced risk of developing Alzheimer's disease (Chang et al. 2016).

However, to have any protective effect, these medications would need to be taken before the disease appears and for a period of at least two years. Taking into account the side effects of NSAIDs, it is not possible to imagine using such anti-inflammatory treatments to prevent Alzheimer's.

Among the natural anti-inflammatories, the top choices should always be the polyunsaturated omega-6s and, more importantly, the omega-3s. These fatty acids can be found in olive oil, flax, walnuts, canola, and high-quality fatty fish.

HYPOVASCULARITY OF THE BRAIN

A reduction of cerebral vascularity can be seen in the brains of Alzheimer's patients. With reduced blood circulation, the body no longer has the ability to eliminate the bulk of the toxins polluting the brain: cellular debris (beta-amyloids), endogenous toxins following chemical reactions, viruses and microbes, chemical medications, heavy metals, mycotoxins caused by fungal infections, and so on. All of these microagressions contribute to breaking through and altering the blood-brain barrier.

We should also note that reduced vascularity is accompanied by a deficiency of oxygen. Oxygen is an essential element for life and supplies energy. The brain is the primary consumer of oxygen; though it represents only 2 percent of our body weight, it consumes 20 percent of the oxygen circulating in the body. A deficit of oxygen will immediately result in destroyed neurons. And as one asphyxia follows another, the neurological aftereffects become increasingly serious.

HEAVY METALS

I think that calling heavy metals "toxic metals" would be more correct. The latter term would cover the entirety of metals and metalloids that are dangerous for health and the environment. They include lead, mercury, arsenic, cadmium, nickel, and bromine, just to mention the most dangerous.

Heavy metals are naturally present in small amounts in nature and in living organisms. But once their quantity exceeds a certain threshold, they become very dangerous, especially because once they are in our bodies, it is very hard to eliminate them.

Aluminum

Around half of all vaccines administered today contain aluminum. Pharmaceutical companies even include a generous amount in the vaccines intended to prevent whooping cough, diphtheria, meningitis, polio, tetanus, and hepatitis A and B in children. (Aluminum adjuvants are not used in live virus vaccines such as the one for measles, mumps, and rubella.)

The typical vaccine regimen for children from two months to sixteen months of age will potentially allow them to receive, in proportion to their weight, aluminum doses that are far higher than the maximum amounts recommended for adults. If we look at the figures provided by the FDA, more than 50 μg per day may not be safe for humans. However, a single vaccine dose can give a baby as much as 650 μg, as pediatrician Robert W. Sears informs us.

The use of vaccines and aluminum in vaccines offers a stunning example of what some see as criminal negligence. In 2010, the vaccine Prevnar 13 was released in the market. This vaccine offers protection against meningitis, pneumonia, and ear infections and is indicated for children from six months to five years old, but it is marketed for adults as well. However, it could also be seen as an illustration of the persistent indifference of the health industry to neurotoxins. In Europe, for example, the agency overseeing medications authorized the vaccine without requiring the manufacturer to use another adjuvant besides aluminum, although substitution is perfectly easy and aluminum is already too widespread in many vaccines.

Vaccine manufacturers as a whole tend to overlook substitutes for aluminum, like calcium phosphate. This compound, which is found naturally in the body, was used in vaccines until the beginning of the 1990s, when it was replaced with aluminum salts, which were less costly. By choosing these salts, pharmaceutical firms gave priority to financial concerns over health concerns, even if they are reluctant to admit it and have a more abstract formulation at hand that shows aluminum offers the "best cost/effectiveness ratio." Alas, this cost/effectiveness ratio doesn't show the human and economical cost of the neurological disorders it may cause, although studies indicating the adverse effects of aluminum continue to accumulate.

Given all the vaccinations and booster shots people are expected to receive, it is easy to see that it is possible for the human brain to contain twenty times more aluminum and other toxic adjuvants than medical science believes healthy.

Aluminum, which is a light metal that can gain entry into the brain quite easily, is frequently found in amyloid plaques. It is a neurotoxin that can be found not just in vaccines but also in municipal water supplies in some areas, medications, cooking utensils, food containers, industrial foods, deodorants, filtered cigarettes, matcha tea, cosmetics, and so forth.

Mercury

Mercury has a strong tendency to collect in the gray matter of the brain, and it is so toxic that there are strict safety measures attached to its use. Even small doses of mercury can alter the human metabolism and nervous system. We are exposed to this heavy metal and its composites when we eat fish that contains high levels of it. The larger and older the fish, the more mercury it contains. Some fish to look out for are tuna, salmon, mackerel, anchovy, sardines, herring, and swordfish.

The mercury we are discussing here is generally methylmercury (the most toxic form of organic mercury), which is produced when microorganisms methylate mercury. But the most significant source of mercury pollution in the body comes from dental amalgams. In this case, we are now talking about elemental mercury. Both methylmercury and elemental mercury can be detected via blood or urine analysis; it is then possible to know from where most of the mercury is coming (fillings or fish).

Under the combined action of saliva and what's called oral galvanism (the different electrical potentials of the various metals used in dental amalgam, resulting in a minute electrical charge), we can see an insidious dissolution of the mercury compounds (and other compounds), leading to a chronic state of poisoning. And mercury poisoning can induce the same symptoms that are characteristic of Alzheimer's disease. It may, in fact, be a contributing factor in Alzheimer's disease.

Mercury, like aluminum, is used in vaccines, in this case as both a preservative and a biocide. Half of the composition of thimerosal, the preservative in many multidose vaccines, is mercury. Thimerosal hasn't been used in children's vaccines since 2001 but is still found in flu vaccines, such as those that were massively prescribed during the 2009–2010 H1N1 swine flu pandemic. Despite the removal of thimerosal from childhood vaccines, many health experts recommended these flu vaccines for children and pregnant women. They maintained that these vaccines were harmless because of the lack of adjuvants, but they remained quite discreet about the fact they contained a substantial amount of mercury, about 45 µg a dose. There seems to be an obvious reluctance on the part of health authorities to turn the spotlight on the injection of millions of doses containing mercury, despite the fact that numerous scientific medical publications have questioned whether it may be a cofactor in the spike of autism and other neurological disorders in the United States. It is now possible to request a flu vaccination from a product without thimerosal.

Arsenic

Arsenic is a semimetallic chemical element, and its toxicity varies depending on the form it takes. Mineral compounds are more toxic than organic ones.

Contaminated water from underground aquifers is one source of exposure. Chronic exposure to high levels of arsenic has been blamed for changes in the brain's executive function, a reduction of mental acuity, and deterioration of verbal abilities, as well as depression.

Cadmium

This heavy metal is concentrated in nickel-cadmium batteries, cigarette smoke, dental amalgams, phosphate fertilizer, silverware polish, and plant protection products (pesticides and fertilizers). It is spread throughout the environment by dirt, then transferred into our crops and foods. It is also found in exhaust emissions, motor oil, enameled pots, porcelain or ceramic dishes, and dyes.

Cadmium is also used in paint, especially yellows and bright reds (the Impressionist painter Monet used cadmium yellow in his paintings of gardens). However, paints today are manufactured in such a way as to greatly reduce the toxic effects of cadmium.

It is difficult for our emunctory organs to eliminate this metal, which is why it can accumulate to dangerous levels in the body. It is typically absorbed into the kidneys, liver, and bones. Cadmium poisoning will cause the same loss of taste and smell that can be found in Alzheimer's disease.

✧✧✧

There are many methods for chelating heavy metals, detoxifying the body, removing blockages that affect the emunctory organs, restoring microflora, and boosting the immune system. All can ease the burden of heavy metals in the body and thereby reduce the risk of Alzheimer's disease.

BIOCIDES AND PESTICIDES

Biocides and pesticides—chemical compounds intended to kill off everything from insects and rodents to bacteria, molds, and mildew—now form a part of our everyday world. They are found in household disinfectants and cleaning products, cosmetic products, lotions, soaps, shampoos, toothpaste, and deodorants. They are used in the manufacture of clothing and leather, building materials, furniture, glue, rubber, and paint. In total, around three hundred biocide formulations are used in the manufacture of several tens of thousands of products. Biocides are even found not just in food containers, where they come in contact with our food, but in foods themselves—namely, in the form of agricultural chemical residues.

Insecticides most often target the nervous system; they are cholinesterase inhibitors. Organophosphates, invented during World War II as a chemical weapon, are acetylcholinesterase inhibitors, meaning that they inhibit the enzyme that breaks down the neurotransmitter acetylcholine. This causes acetylcholine to accumulate on the synapses and, after a brief period of stimulation, block the transmission of nerve impulses.

Given those mechanisms, it should not be surprising to hear that chronic exposure to pesticides has cumulatively toxic effects on the central nervous system and can be linked to the development of Alzheimer's disease (Yan et al. 2016).

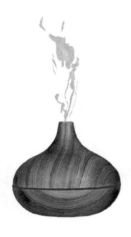

9

Additional Risk Factors and Considerations

Knowledge Is Power

WE KNOW TODAY that it is possible to grow old in good health, without suffering any symptoms of Alzheimer's disease, or delaying them long enough that they appear only at a very late stage of life. Moreover, we can achieve this, without medications, simply by applying some fairly simple preventive measures.

While there is still no absolute certainty about why the disease occurs in some people and not in others, it has been proved that prevention (primarily through an organic diet) can delay its onset by several years. The primary risk factors are perfectly identifiable. According to a 2011 study by Deborah Barnes and Kristine Yaffe, published in *Lancet Neurology*, approximately 19 percent of Alzheimer's cases can be linked to a low level of education, 14 percent to tobacco use, 13 percent to lack of physical activity, 11 percent to depression, 5 percent to high blood pressure, 2 percent to obesity, and 2 percent to diabetes.

We should not look at prevention as a series of things we cannot do but as a list of good resolutions that we can adjust on a daily basis.

AGE

Alzheimer's disease is estimated to be present in 5 to 7 percent of individuals over the age of sixty-five. The frequency of the disease practically doubles every five years after the age of seventy, with a clear majority of women affected. The disease affects one out of five people in the population over the age of eighty-five.

As it happens, the number of people older than eighty-five continues to increase with the lengthening life spans and the graying of the population, which is why Alzheimer's disease has become a veritable public health problem.

SEX

The disease is more frequent in men under the age of sixty-five, but this predominance reverses after that age, which has led to the assumption that hormonal factors connected with menopause may be to blame in older populations. To mitigate the effects of the hormonal deficiency caused by menopause, it has been suggested that women replace these missing hormones, using what is known as hormone replacement therapy (HRT). Unfortunately, chemical HRT has been implicated as a possible factor in 40 percent of breast cancers. My advice would be to use natural therapies instead (diet, herbs, essential oils, homeopathy).

We should note that menopausal women who do not adopt some sort of hormone replacement program are four times more likely to develop Alzheimer's disease than those who do.

LEVEL OF EDUCATION

The frequency of the disease is higher among the individuals with a lesser degree of education. On the other hand, the higher the level of education, the less we see Alzheimer's disease; the intensive stimulation of the brain during adolescence and young adulthood strengthens the neurons and their connections, making it possible to expand, in some way, the capital of cognitive reserve.

The brain, endowed with an extreme level of plasticity, is not a rigid organ. Education appears to increase the capacity for plasticity by a set of intellectual stimulations that allow brain performance to be optimized by the recruitment of other regions of the brain.

CARDIOVASCULAR RISK FACTORS

Cardiovascular risk factors include high blood pressure, diabetes, high cholesterol and/or triglyceride levels, a sedentary lifestyle, being overweight or obese, the use of tobacco, and a medical history of stroke.

The brain has poor tolerance for increased pressure in the veins that irrigate it. High blood pressure is responsible for poor blood circulation. Over time, the oxygenation of the brain lessens in quality, and cerebral function is disturbed, with possible infarction. Unstabilized high blood pressure multiplies the risk of dementia six times.

The Cholesterol Paradox

Many people have high cholesterol levels but don't have any cardiovascular problems, whereas many others who have normal cholesterol suffer from heart disease. Here is a paradoxical fact: a low rate of cholesterol is associated with cognitive decline. When total cholesterol falls below 1.5 g/L, the risk of cerebral atrophy increases. This may be because cholesterol is a key element of the cellular membranes (and especially the cerebral cells).

Conversely, treatment of high blood pressure reduces the risk of Alzheimer's disease because of the drop in arterial pressure. This is why monitoring blood pressure is essential in the preventive treatment of Alzheimer's.

MEDICAL HISTORY OF SKULL/BRAIN TRAUMA

A major trauma or repeated traumas (as in the case of boxers) encourages expression of Alzheimer's disease because of the neuron loss the trauma causes. The most demonstrative example of this would be the boxer Muhammad Ali.

SLEEP APNEA

Sleep apnea is a disorder characterized by repeated temporary cessations in breathing while sleeping. It affects a large number of people and represents a serious risk factor for cognitive decline.

Sleep tests make it possible to score patients on the apnea-hypopnea index (AHI), a scale that corresponds to the number of times breathing stops during one hour of sleep. A normal AHI score is less than 5, and the objective target is 0. People with sleep apnea may have as many as 100 stops per hour.

Many patients do not know they have sleep apnea. They don't notice the breathing stops, but their spouse or partner does. It is possible to detect the condition at home with the help of a portable testing device. In the event that sleep apnea is suspected, an ear-nose-throat exam will be called for and a sleep study, called a polysomnography, will be undertaken to get a diagnosis. Even so, the majority of people who suffer from this disorder are not diagnosed.

Treatment for sleep apnea primarily involves weight loss but may also include using continuous positive airway pressure (CPAP) machine at night, which will provide constant pulmonary ventilation.

GOOD SLEEP

There are two distinct aspects to sleep, which, though obvious, are often overlooked: quantitative and qualitative.

The quantitative aspect is simply duration. Seven to eight hours of sleep are necessary. Sleep can be disturbed by stress, conflict, rumination, or anxiety, which can be treated in the same way as stress. Herbs, homeopathy, and acupuncture can all provide valuable assistance.

The qualitative aspect is determined by digestion. When digestion is working properly, sleep will be of good quality, and upon waking up (after seven or eight hours of it), we feel fit as a fiddle.

Sleep has two essential roles. First, it permits physical recuperation after a day of activity. This is the period during which the metabolism repairs itself. Second, sleep allows memorization. This is the period during which the brain puts away the information it took in during the day. It classifies and compares each piece and creates analogies. This is how we can wake up in the morning with the answer to a problem we were not able to solve the day before.

A good night's sleep includes a phase of deep sleep when neurons shrink and the interstitial spaces—the gaps between brain tissues—widen. This allows cerebrospinal fluid to circulate better and allows for the better elimination of toxins, such as excess beta-amyloids, through the blood-brain barrier. A good night's sleep also strengthens neurogenesis in the hippocampus.

Down with Sleeping Pills

Millions of medications against insomnia are consumed on a daily basis in Western countries! Benzodiazepines, for example, are often prescribed for their sleep-inducing effects, but they produce numerous side effects, the most frequent of which is sedation. The symptoms include drowsiness, light-headedness, difficulty concentrating, slurred speech, memory lapses, mental confusion, and problems with balance and coordination. Elderly patients are the most sensitive to this kind of medication, and they are the ones for whom it is most often prescribed.

The other major perverse effect of this kind of sleeping pill is its addictive nature. After using it for only several weeks, psychological and physical dependence becomes established, and the body will need the medication to function normally. At the same time, the sleep-inducing effect diminishes after several weeks. However, insomniacs continue to use the medication to avoid withdrawal symptoms such as hypersensitivity, muscle tics, and other unpleasant sensations.

In addition to these numerous side effects, the sleep induced by sleeping pills in not a natural sleep. The structure of sleep becomes altered, and the two phases that are most important, paradoxical sleep (a.k.a. REM sleep) and deep sleep, are sharply reduced.

All these negative side effects should motivate us to look more to natural solutions to treat our sleeping problems. Melatonin is one such remedy.

The Utility of Dreams

An absence of dreams could represent a predisposition to Alzheimer's and the sign of a poorly functioning brain. Furthermore, it could signal a flawed integration of the data recorded over the day. The role of dreaming is to digest the events that occurred during the day, emotional stressors, and a whole set of irritations. The role played by dreams makes it possible to file the collected information into our various memories and to connect these bits of information to other elements that have already been integrated in the hard disk that makes up our brain. This is how we create associations between ideas and deductions based on facts in order to analyze the experiences we've lived through. The absence of dreaming means that this integration is not taking place and would explain in particular the troubles that Alzheimer's patients have with recent memory, as these experiences are no longer being recorded.

DRUGS

Regular use of drugs like cocaine, heroin, and opium can cause psychotic mental disorders, apathetic and catatonic states, and troubles with attention, memory, concentration, and movement coordination.

Cannabis, too, can contribute to memory problems. The naturally occurring, biologically active compounds found in cannabis are called cannabinoids. The two main ones are tetrahydrocannabinol (THC) and cannabidiol (CBD). (It is only THC, and not CBD, that has psychoactive properties.) There are numerous cannabinoid receptors in the brain. While it causes relaxation, induces a feeling of euphoria and well-being, and alters perception, cannabis can also reduce the connections between the neurons of the hippocampus, which can make it hard for consumers to concentrate.

Cannabis for Alzheimer's Treatment?

The primary domain for the medical use of cannabis is for palliative care. Specific studies have been made on the effect of cannabinoids on Alzheimer's disease, but only in mice. Looking ahead, we know that CBD has an anti-inflammatory and antioxidant action in the brain; it could perhaps stimulate neurogenesis in the hippocampus, thus fighting against Alzheimer's disease. THC, meanwhile, could inhibit the accumulation of amyloid plaques.

By virtue of its amnesia-inducing effect, THC, in the proper dosage, could also have a positive effect by erasing painful or traumatic memories.

It has been observed in those who consume cannabis on a daily basis that two cerebral zones are reduced in size: the hippocampus, involved in the regulation of memory, and the amygdala, involved in emotions and tendencies to aggression.

ELECTROMAGNETIC WAVES

The electromagnetic waves of radio frequencies pass invisibly through the air. Emitted mainly by cell phones or relay masts, they make it possible for us to transmit information with our electronic devices. But some studies have blamed them for various pathologies: headaches, sleep troubles, memory problems, tinnitus, and so on.

A wide variety of electromagnetic rays exist, distinguished by the energies they carry and their possible interactions with biological structures. These rays are divided into two complementary models, moving either as electromagnetic waves (wavelike model) or as a flow of photons (corpuscular model).

Cell phones, Wi-Fi, baby monitors, antennas, and other devices that emit electromagnetic rays all provide great help every day and are so commonplace that we pay barely any attention to them. There is good reason for this; the waves they emit are invisible, inaudible, and undetectable. But could they have an effect on our bodies nevertheless? The tortures suffered by individuals who have become supersensitive to these electromagnetic fields shows us that the answer is yes.

Wireless transmission technologies could not exist without relay masts, which are currently suspected of having adverse effects on human health, including headaches, sleep disorders, tinnitus, and even Alzheimer's disease. While it is true that these symptoms often have a multitude of factors as their origin, several studies have shown that the prevalence of headaches; problems affecting memory, sleep, and concentration; dizzy spells; trembling; and depressive states is higher among people living close to relay masts, such as those found in cell towers.

THE MODERN DIET

Diet is an important factor—perhaps the most important factor—in many of the leading causes of death, like cardiovascular diseases, cancers, metabolic storage diseases, and neurodegenerative diseases. Our modern diet is strongly condemned because it is so far removed from the ancestral diet for which our body seems to have been genetically programmed.

For millions of years, humans consumed a natural diet of mainly raw foods, similar to that of wild animals. Following the laws of evolution, our digestive mucins and enzymes are adapted to that diet.

If we were to recapitulate the great transformations that distinguish the modern diet from the ancestral diet, we could identify six:

1. The poor nutritional quality of the food due to the perverse effects of intensive agriculture and factory farming, with pesticides and chemical fertilizers that impoverish the soils and consequently the plants that grow in them. These plants are deficient in essential nutrients like calcium, magnesium, trace elements, and so forth.

2. The consumption of domesticated grains that cause gluten intolerance, which then adversely affects the neurotransmitters. (We'll discuss gluten intolerance later in this chapter.)

3. The consumption of animal milks and their derivatives; casein, which makes up 85 percent of the protein found in milk, is a phosphoprotein (a protein with a phosphate group attached). The excess phosphorus destroys calcium, which is essential for the construction of neurotransmitters.

4. The cooking of many substances, which creates degenerative products.

5. The preparation of oils.
6. Excessive use of salt.

Excessive Salt

Sodium works in tandem with potassium in the body. A balance is constantly maintained between these two substances: when sodium levels rise, potassium levels fall, and vice versa.

The problem is that our modern Western diet has way too much sodium, with an almost systematic addition of salt in all industrially prepared foods: premade dishes, sauces, canned goods, deli meats, and so forth. The current salt-to-potassium (Na:K) ratio in the diet of developed countries is on the order of 2:4. Our prehistoric ancestors' diet had an Na:K ratio of 0:1! So it is very desirable to start by reducing our salt consumption as excessive salt causes water retention, which, in turn, causes smothered and drowned cells to break down and die.

A poor Na:K ratio causes:

+ High blood pressure
+ Stroke
+ Diabetes (through its effect on glucose)
+ Weight gain
+ General and cerebral aging

A good Na:K ratio is essential for the conduction of nerve impulses along the axons of nerve cells. In fact, the passage of nerve impulses is determined by the electrical potential difference existing on either side of the cellular membrane. This difference of potential is realized by the sodium and potassium balance on each side of the membrane; in other words, the Na:K ratio is responsible for the depolarization of the membrane and the good circulation of nerve impulses.

To lower this Na:K ratio, the logical step is to limit your

consumption of sodium as well as to increase your intake of potassium. Foods rich in potassium include dried fruits, oleaginous fruits, raw vegetables, bananas, apricots, fruit juices, and so on.

Excessive Sugar

Refined sugar is endemic in modern food, in candies, cakes, pastries, jams, chocolate, soda, and sweetened beverages. And while sugar is an extract of natural products (sugarcane, beets), its refinement, with the numerous chemical manipulations that involves, makes it a degraded and toxic product if eaten regularly and in excessive quantities.

Once it is metabolized inside the body, dietary sugar causes a substantial rise in blood sugar (hyperglycemia), which stimulates us, making us very active, if not excited and nervous. When faced with heightened blood sugar levels, the pancreas releases a large amount of insulin to make the amount of sugar circulating in the blood drop.

This doesn't restore normal blood sugar levels, though. Instead, blood sugar levels continue to drop (hypoglycemia), causing dizziness (and a risk of falling), fatigue, a general feeling of malaise, and a confused state. Chronic hypoglycemia is very detrimental to the brain because sugar is essential for neuronal activity. As it happens, the brain possesses only a few seconds' worth of sugar reserves! Repeated drops in blood sugar contribute to the destruction of neurons and all cerebral functions.

Gluten Intolerance

Banned by the hypotoxic (Seignalet) and paleo diets, gluten is a group of proteins that are present in grains. It is gluten that makes it possible to turn flour into bread. It is gluten that gives bread dough its resistance and elasticity and allows it to rise by means of fermentation and heat.

The term *gluten* actually denotes a blend of two protein families: prolamins and glutenins.

Some prolamins, including gliadin (found in wheat, spelt, and kamut), secalin (found in rye), and hordein (found in barley), are toxic for people with celiac disease. Prolamins can also be found in other grains, like oats (avenin), maize (zein), sorghum (kafirin), rice (orzenin), and millet (panicin), but these latter do not appear to be toxic for people with celiac disease, although there is still a substantial debate about oats.

Glutenins are also toxic for people who suffer from celiac disease, but to a lesser degree. In total there are more than fifty protein residues of gluten that are identified as toxic for celiac patients.

Poor Absorption of Gluten and Celiac Disease

According to the most recent studies on celiac disease, the mechanism responsible for it is the following: During digestion, enzymes carve apart proteins into smaller pieces. In the case of gluten, this carving is incomplete, and nondigested protein fragments end up in the small intestine. This results in an increase of intestinal permeability—it could be that the gluten itself is responsible for this increased permeability—that makes it possible for these fragments to travel through the normally tight junctions. These fragments then run into an enzyme called tissue transglutaminase that slightly alters their structure. These altered proteins now have an antigenic potential—which is to say, that in predisposed individuals, they will start an immune reaction and trigger the production of IgA antibodies that target the gliadin of the gluten and the tissue transglutaminase. This reaction causes an inflammatory response that results in destruction of the intestinal villi in the small intestine, causing partial destruction of the intestinal wall. This causes improper absorption and therefore serious deficiencies in certain nutrients (mineral salts, vitamins).

When gluten is no longer being ingested, the antibodies gradually disappear. After a period of several months, the intestine heals and the patient goes into remission. However, the presence of even the smallest gluten molecule in the body will retrigger the attack, targeting the intestinal mucous membrane and thus the patient.

Where Is Gluten Found?

Industrial bakeries often add substantial amounts of gluten to the flour they use in their products. In times past, the traditional method for activating gluten was kneading. Today, a substantially higher amount of gluten is needed in the flour to compensate for the fact that, instead of kneading by hand, current industrial procedures require the dough to be kneaded mechanically, partially baked, and then frozen, followed by storage and transport to the place where it will be thawed and then finish baking.

Gluten is present in many products where you might expect to find it, such as beer and soy sauce, but is also used as a stabilizing agent and thickener in the most unexpected food products, such as ice cream and ketchup. These hidden sources of gluten can pose a problem for people suffering from celiac disease as well as those who have a degree of sensitivity to gluten. A rigorous monitoring of gluten content is therefore necessary for the certification of foods that are suitable for consumption by these individuals.

Gluten is also used in the manufacture of pharmaceutical products (nonprescription medications, mouthwashes, herbal health products, food supplements, adhesive bandages and dressings), all kinds of cosmetic and personal care products (lipsticks, lip glosses, ointments, toothpastes, hair care and skin care products, and so on). It is found in farm animal feed and pet food (to increase their protein content), pet shampoos, modeling clay for children (like Play-Doh), and so forth.

Symptoms of Gluten Intolerance

Gluten intolerance is hard to diagnose because its symptoms are varied and not specifically connected to this disease. Furthermore, the symptoms differ depending on whether the sufferer is a child or an adult.

In infants, the symptoms can appear several weeks after the introduction of flour into their diet, and they are highly varied: chronic diarrhea, hypertrophy, weight loss, slowed or even halted growth, vomiting, and so forth. In adults, symptoms include gastrointestinal disorders (stomach pain, difficult digestion, diarrhea, soft stools, gastroesophageal reflux disease, vomiting, gastric stasis, bloating), joint problems, neurological disorders, dermatological problems, stomach problems, numerous deficiencies due to poor nutrient absorption, anemia, osteoporosis, chronic fatigue, and so on.

People suffering from gluten intolerance can spend years getting medical attention before the diagnosis is made. Untreated celiac disease not only causes a reduced quality of life but also increases the risk of intestinal lymphomas and a shortened life span. It is also associated with a number of other autoimmune diseases, such as type 1 diabetes, Hashimoto's thyroiditis, gluten ataxia, psoriasis, vitiligo, rheumatoid arthritis, ankylosing spondylitis, inflammatory intestinal diseases (Crohn's disease), systemic lupus erythematosus, autoimmune hepatitis, dermatitis herpetiformis, primary sclerosing cholangitis, and so on.

Intestinal Hyperpermeability (Leaky Gut)

The dismantling of the tight junctions of the intestinal wall causes hyperpermeability of the intestinal wall, a condition also known as leaky gut. Gluten (whether or not in the presence of celiac disease) and lipopolysaccharides (LPSs) arising from a chronic bacterial colonization of the small intestine would seem to be the primary culprits. Hyperpermeability of the intestinal wall allows the increased entrance into the bloodstream of substances that should practically never gain access (microorganisms; bacterial toxins, primarily LPSs; partially digested foods). These substances stimulate the immune system and, based on the individual's genetic predispositions, cause a variety of medical problems.

A 2011 study suggests that changes in intestinal wall permeability can in some cases be responsible for the development of:

+ Autoimmune diseases
+ Cancers, such as glioma (cancer of the brain or spinal cord), breast cancer, ovarian cancer, pancreatic cancer, prostate cancer, adenocarcinoma of the lung, hepatocellular carcinoma in the presence of a hepatitis C infection, acute nonlymphocytic leukemia, diffuse large B-cell lymphoma, and acute myeloid leukemia
+ Nervous system disorders, such as multiple sclerosis, schizophrenia, chronic inflammatory demyelinating polyradiculoneuropathy (CIDP), inflammatory optic neuritis, allergies, infections, and asthma

Gluten ataxia is an autoimmune disease triggered by ingesting gluten. It causes damage to the cerebellum, the balance center of the brain that controls coordination and complex movements like walking, speaking, and swallowing. Early diagnosis and treatment with a gluten-free diet can improve ataxia and prevent its progression. The effectiveness of the treatment depends on how long the patient has been suffering from ataxia, as the death of the neurons in the cerebellum following exposure to gluten is irreversible.

Diagnosing Gluten Intolerance

To make a diagnosis of gluten intolerance, it is necessary to look for the specific antibodies of the disease (anti-transglutaminase antibodies) in a blood sample. In the event of a positive result, an endoscopy should follow with samples (biopsies) from the upper part of the small intestine (duodenum). Last, the health care professional should determine whether a remission occurs after the patient has been put on a gluten-free diet. In fact, the effectiveness of a gluten-free diet on the improvement of disease symptoms and the restoration of the intestinal villi (after twelve to eighteen months) confirms the gluten intolerance diagnosis.

A Gluten-Free Diet

Logically, all patients who are victims of gluten intolerance should be able to easily abstain from ingesting it. But here we find a veritable mafia that makes a profit on it. Fortunately, with the growing popularity of healthy and organic foods, it is now possible to find perfectly good grain products certified to be gluten-free.

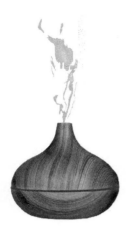

10

The Body's Five Protective Barriers

And What Happens When They Rupture

AS A WAY TO PROTECT us from aggressive foreign elements and antigens, our bodies have five filters at their disposal:

- ✦ The intestinal barrier
- ✦ The reticuloendothelial system barrier
- ✦ The vascular endothelium
- ✦ Blood cells
- ✦ The blood-brain barrier

THE INTESTINAL BARRIER

Our intestines are an ecosystem in their own right, one that rests on a functional tripod: the intestinal microbiome (intestinal flora), the intestinal mucous membrane, and the intestinal immune system, which act together in synergy and symbiosis. This functional tripod takes care of the completion of the digestive process, assimilation, the recognition of nutrients, and the creation of our "identity" (intestinal immunity).

The intestines are the primary immune organ of our bodies. In fact, approximately 60 percent of the body's immune cells are located in our intestinal mucous membrane.

The intestines also house an impressive microbial population, with one hundred billion beneficial and physiologically necessary bacteria, located primarily in the colon. Unfortunately, daily exposure to chemical products, pollutants, harmful bacteria in drinking water, antibiotic residues in food, medications, refined foods, and other harmful factors, combined with a poor diet and high levels of stress, can ravage the balance and effectiveness of the intestinal microbiome. An imbalanced microbiome is the origin of the proliferation of harmful and pathogenic microorganisms.

The functional effectiveness of the intestinal ecosystem is connected to the synergy of its three components. Any disturbance of the ecosystem can distort the recognition of a food by the intestinal immune system, which then leads to a food intolerance. This process often plays a role in the creation of functional or pathological problems and should be taken into account when offering dietary advice.

The intestinal ecosystem is therefore essential to our overall state of health. The intestinal microbiome is the most vulnerable foundational element of this functional synergy. Any phenomenon that disturbs this microbiome will work against the assimilation-absorption process and have an adverse effect on our nutritional status.

The management and protection of this ecosystem is achieved through rebalancing and supporting the beneficial microorganisms in the intestines. This can be done using specific food supplements: probiotics and prebiotics.

The Intestinal Microbiome

Every individual has their own intestinal microbiome profile; this profile is unique both qualitatively and quantitatively. It is somewhat the same as a bacterial fingerprint. Many factors, including how we were born (natural or Caesarian), whether we were nursed by our mother, the variety and quality of our diet, our geographical surroundings, hygienic conditions, vaccinations (multiple or early), gastric acidity, interactions between bacteria, antibodies, mucus, and so forth, have an influence on the diversity, composition, and metabolic activity of our intestinal microflora.

The microorganisms that make up our intestinal microbiome include more than five hundred different species of bacteria, divided into little niche environments all along the digestive tract. There are very few in the stomach (too acidic) and the duodenum. They are much more present in the small intestine and even more so in the colon.

The microbiome therefore consists of colonies, and it is their balance that ensures optimal function. Their mission is to coexist, to prevent potentially harmful strains from developing, and to work together to promote good intestinal functioning.

As a whole, the intestinal microbiome is very sensitive to change.

The Intestinal Mucous Membrane

The second element of the tripod, the intestinal mucous membrane, is an extraordinarily well-crafted protective coating for the intestines. It is renewed on a constant basis: all its constituent cells (enterocytes) are renewed every three weeks. The mucous membrane cells are connected to each other by complex conjunctive fibers. When these junctions are altered, they come apart and allow larger molecules to pass between them and into the bloodstream (hyperpermeability). These larger molecules are often undesirable and toxic elements such as germs and viruses. This causes dysbiosis—disruption of the microbiome's homeostasis.

Various fuels are required to support the tissues of the mucous membrane: polyunsaturated fatty acids to form the cellular membrane, proteins (glutamine, arginine) for cell renewal, and antioxidants for cellular protection. All these nutrients work together to maintain the vitality and proper functioning of this mucous membrane.

The Intestinal Immune System

The immune system consists of a coordinated group of identification and defense elements that govern the differentiation of "self" from "non-self." Those elements considered "non-self," like viruses, bacteria, parasites, and certain foreign molecules or particles, are neutralized.

The intestinal tract is the largest body surface that is exposed to non-self pollutants. The intestinal immune system has two essential, and seemingly contradictory, means at its disposal for protecting the intestinal tract and, thus, the entire body. The first is an activation of immune reaction: the manufacture of antibodies that fight off danger-ous bacteria, viruses, and parasites in the digestive tract. The second involves almost total neutralization of immune reactions, in this case the presence of foreign food proteins. This phenomenon grants us what is known as "oral tolerance" (food tolerance).

Together, these two functions allow us to assimilate all the nutri-ents we need to support our bodies while also arming ourselves against any harmful invader.

The Direct Brain-Intestines Relationship

Structurally and functionally, the intestinal nervous system (or enteric nervous system) and the brain resemble one another. They use the same structure of sensory and motor neurons, the same circuits for processing information, the same glial cells, and the same neurotrans-mitters (acetylcholine, noradrenaline, dopamine, and serotonin). The intestines, in fact, contain more than one hundred million neurons, release at least twenty types of neurotransmitters identi-cal to those found in the brain, and produce the bulk of the body's immune cells.

The combination of the two phenomena of dysbiosis and intestinal inflammation activates the intestinal nervous system, causing the release of neurotransmitters that activate nerve cells in the various regions of the brain and spawning metabolic disturbances like diabetes and obesity.

Rebuilding the Intestinal Barrier

When the intestinal barrier—the microbiome, mucous membrane, or immune function in the intestines—is weakened, we can rebuild it via several methods.

Supplementation

L-glutamine is the most abundant amino acid in our blood and muscles. It plays a role in the synthesis of proteins, immune protection, ensuring the integrity of the intestinal wall, and the acid-alkaline balance (pH) of the body. It is an important nutrient for proper gastrointestinal function. It is the preferred fuel of enterocytes. It plays a major role in the maintenance of the intestinal mucous membrane by encouraging the repair of the epithelium, thereby taking part in the restoration of the intestinal barrier.

Other food supplements that can be taken in combination with L-glutamine to restore the intestinal barrier include:

+ L-methione, which acts synergistically with L-glutamine
+ Gamma-oryzanol, a natural component of rice bran, which has numerous beneficial effects on the gastrointestinal mucous membrane
+ Turmeric, which has anti-inflammatory effects and can inhibit and destroy *H. pylori* bacteria, which are responsible for the majority of gastric and duodenal ulcers
+ Glutathione, a major antioxidant that reduces the inflammation

caused by gastritis, stomach ulcers, pancreatitis, and intestinal swelling, including colon ulcers and Crohn's disease

Healing Lesions

Inflammation and irritation in the intestinal mucous membrane degrades its ability to function as an effective barrier. Targeting those irritations, or lesions, can improve its function.

Thanks to its alkalizing mineral composition, green clay helps buffer excess acidity and regulate acid-alkaline balance. It is also used for its detoxifying, absorbent, healing, and remineralizing properties. It carpets the gastrointestinal mucous membrane, protects it, helps heal wounds (irritation, ulcerous lesions), and absorbs the gas and toxins present in the digestive tract.

Zinc citrate, because of its citrate form, has a polarity (electromagnetic charge) that is biocompatible with that of the small intestine, making it easier for the body to assimilate. This is an essential nutrient for the intestinal mucous membrane; it plays a part in healing internal injuries and has an anti-inflammatory effect. Zinc citrate works as a major buffer in the entire body, thereby helping to maintain its acid-alkaline balance.

Spirulina contains a treasure trove of nutrients in a very small package: it is 70 percent protein and contains all the essential amino acids. It is extremely high in iron, vitamins, and gamma-linolenic acid (an anti-inflammatory fatty acid). Spirulina is also an excellent source of chlorophyll, which has a healing and purifying effect on the gastrointestinal mucous membrane.

Prebiotics and Probiotics

Prebiotics are substances that promote the growth of beneficial bacteria in the intestinal microbiome. Probiotics are living microorganisms that, when consumed in sufficient quantities and with a good combination of strains, encourage the development and balance of the intestinal microflora.

Not all probiotic bacterial strains have the same properties. Some contribute to rebalancing our intestinal flora, while others improve transit, encourage the absorption of minerals and vitamins, or strengthen the immune system. The effects of a probiotic are therefore dependent on the bacterial strain as well as the number of organisms, which, to be active, must consist of a billion bacteria at minimum.

Acacia fibers are a good source of roughage with prebiotic effects; they improve the production of butyrate and propionate, are very easily digested, and make better intestinal transit possible. Fibregum, a prebiotic supplement made from acacia sap, is a good source of that fiber. It permits better intestinal transit and strengthens the synergistic activity of the beneficial bacteria.

THE RETICULOENDOTHELIAL SYSTEM BARRIER

The reticuloendothelial system (RES) barrier consists of lymphocytes produced by stem cells of the lymphoid tissue following the invasion of the body by antigens (foreign bodies). These cells will transform into B and T lymphocytes as well as plasmocytes with immune properties.

The RES corresponds to a group of cells spread throughout the body, most especially in certain support tissues such as the conjunctive tissue but also in the lymphatic ganglia, the liver (Kupfer cells), bone marrow, the spleen (where the cells are organized into a network, giving rise to the prefix *reticulo-*), tonsils, Peyer's patches, the appendix, and the pulmonary alveoli.

All the cells of the reticuloendothelial system possess an identical nature: they are stem cells with the ability to transform themselves, and thereby they give birth to most of the blood cells and, more particularly, to the monocytes that change into macrophages, intended to absorb and catabolize elements that are foreign to the body.

THE VASCULAR ENDOTHELIUM

Two structures form the framework of vascular vessels: collagen and elastic (or connective) tissue. Sulfur, copper, zinc, silicon, and manganese are the constitutive elements of connective tissue, which is composed of three types of protein. One of those protein groups plays the role of a bonding agent: the proteoglycans—namely, chondroitin sulfate and keratin.

The bulk of phagocytic cells (polymorphonuclear leukocytes, macrophages, and monocytes) lodge themselves in the vascular walls and connective tissue. These are antigen-presenting cells, similar to the dendritic cells of the intestinal mucosa and the astrocytes of the blood-brain barrier.

The vascular endothelium forms a cellular barrier between the tissues and blood. It is a key factor in the regulation of vessel tone and structure. In response to various stimuli, the endothelial cells are capable of synthetizing regulator molecules. Some mechanical or physiological conditions are able to hamper this function, causing what is referred to as an endothelial dysfunction. It is characterized by a flaw of the endothelium-dependent vasodilation caused by the reduced availability of vasodilating factors, such as nitric oxide, and an increase of endothelial activation.

BLOOD CELLS

Our blood cells are composed of monocytes and B lymphocytes (or B cells). The monocytes become macrophages, and the B lymphocytes produce antibodies.

THE BLOOD-BRAIN BARRIER

One system escapes the initial attack of antigens: the central nervous system, which consists of the brain, spinal cord, and peripheral nervous system. The central nervous system is essential for the transmission of nerve impulses and in this respect is protected by the blood-brain barrier.

The complex functions of the brain are connected to very sensitive biochemical and electrochemical processes, which are only able to occur within an internal environment of homeostatic balance, from which all disturbance has been removed. This is why variations in blood pH (a measure of the acid-alkaline balance) cannot help but have repercussions on the brain. The same can be said for variations in the concentration of potassium, which can disrupt the potential of the nerve cells' membrane.

The essential elements of the blood-brain barrier are endothelial cells and astrocytes. The junctions between these cells are tighter than those between other types of cells. The protection offered by the blood-brain barrier is so effective that even many medications cannot pass through it.

Astrocytes

Of an exclusively perivascular topography organized into a grid, the astrocytes form the real blood-brain barrier of the central nervous system. Their role is to protect neurons from foreign substances capable of entering the brain. To achieve this, the astrocytes form an airtight epithelium that carpets the cerebral ventricles and the ependymal canal of the spinal cord.

In addition to their protective duties, astrocytes play a major role in the maintenance of neuronal synapses and in the myelination processes of the nerve fibers. They produce, among other neurotropic factors, nerve growth. They form the primary site for capturing the glucose necessary for neuron activity, thanks to the presence in their membrane of glucose transporters (GLUT1 and GLUT2). They also play a role in the recapture of neurotransmitters and in breaking them down, and they take part in the regulation of extracellular pH thanks to the Na+/K+/H+ channels (proton pumps) and calcium channels.

Without astrocytes, neurons could not develop or propagate nerve impulses, the vascular endothelium would be incapable of ensuring the isolation of the central nervous system, and oligodendrocytes would be unable to divide and assume their functions. Good relations between astrocytes and neurons are the guarantee of cerebral balance.

The Microglial Cells

These cells are embryologically derived from blood monocytes that have crossed through the blood-brain barrier. Therefore, like monocytes, they possess phagocytic properties and mobility. Microglial cells are sometimes perivascular, like astrocytes, and sometimes simply located in the proximity of the vessels. A good number of glial cells are antigen-presenting. They collect in the regions of dead or altered neurons, such as those found in Parkinson's disease, Alzheimer's disease, and multiple sclerosis.

The Rupture of the Blood-Brain Barrier

As is the case for the intestinal epithelium, it is the accumulation of all and sundry foreign substances or the presence of a superantigen that causes a hypersensitive reaction and the appearance of circulating immune complexes (CICs), which are harmful to the vascular walls of the blood-brain barrier.

The incessant flood of antigens promotes the deposit of CICs and worsens the calcium inhibitor mechanism. The latter will eventually invert, causing a blockage of the potassium channels with a rupture of the blood-brain barrier through an ischemic mechanism responsible for causing problems with neuronal structures.

The progressive rupture of the blood-brain barrier under the attack of antigens is proportional to the seriousness of the oxidizing stress, which starts with an attack on the axons of the peripheral nerves, followed by the axons of the nerves of the central nervous system, before reaching the neuronal bodies.

Depending on an antigen's affinity with this or that receptor (or neurotransmission path), the result will be one of three diseases:

+ Amyotrophic lateral sclerosis, or Lou Gehrig's disease, associated with medulla nicotinic receptors
+ Alzheimer's disease, associated with cortical nicotinic receptors
+ Parkinson's disease, associated with dopaminergic receptors

Influential Factors in a Blood-Brain Barrier Rupture

These factors can be superimposed on the factors that generate oxidizing stress. They depend upon:

+ The nature of the antigen; for example, the hepatitis B virus, Epstein-Barr virus, and cytomegalovirus have the singular feature of being persistent and are considered to be superantigens
+ The cumulative dose of the antigens
+ The duration of exposure to the antigen

Oral contraceptives, which cause reduced activity of the enzymes that metabolize foreign substances (cytochrome P450 enzymes), boost the chances of a blood-brain barrier rupture. Hormone replacement therapy and anti-inflammatory steroids likewise contribute to the breakdown of the blood-brain barrier.

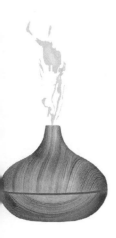

11

Neuroplasticity

Caring for the Brain

IT WAS LONG BELIEVED that nerve cells were incapable of reproduction. It was thought that we started life with a certain neuron capital at our disposal and that it was impossible to regenerate or restore neurons. But we know today that, under certain conditions, neurogenesis—the development of new nerve cells—is possible.

The brain, which consists of neural networks, is constantly reinventing itself. Everything we experience and everything we learn changes our neuronal wiring. When we learn, when we imagine, we create new zones of junction between neurons (the synapses); this process strengthens some networks, and we lose others. These changes comprise what is known as cerebral plasticity.

Intellectual practice develops certain parts of the cortex, which could be likened to a veritable cerebral GPS. Similarly, after a lesion (stroke), the brain renews itself by finding alternative paths around the damaged tissue. To compensate for the lost neurons, regions that specialize in other functions will supply them. But it is obvious that the older we get, the more our capacity for brain plasticity will lessen.

Two concepts have been identified that make up the heart of this cerebral plasticity: the cerebral reserve and the cognitive reserve. These concepts make it possible to understand why cognitive stimulation throughout our entire life is a providential path for preventing Alzheimer's disease.

THE CEREBRAL RESERVE

The cerebral reserve represents a passive quantity connected to the structural elements of the brain, such as its size and weight. This includes the mass of the neurons and especially the volume of connections between them (synaptic connections) and the dendrites surrounding the neural nuclei, the "dendritic trees." The cerebral reserve represents the available brain structures that we can draw upon as needed.

THE COGNITIVE RESERVE

The cognitive reserve is an active process of neuroplasticity. This process is an adaptive cerebral flexibility—which is to say, our capacity for optimizing our cognitive performance. This optimization can be the result of drawing on other cerebral regions or even simply making use of new cognitive therapies or alternatives developed from the habitually utilized cognitive resources.

It has been widely observed that plasticity can be developed even among the elderly. It is possible that supporting brain plasticity could delay the expression of the deficits caused by Alzheimer's disease for several years. This on its own already constitutes immense progress in our approach to treating the disease.

BUILDING THE COGNITIVE RESERVE

Scientists have talked about the concept of a brain reserve (a.k.a. cerebral reserve) for decades, but in 2012, American neuroscientist Yaakov Stern proposed separating the idea of a passive cerebral reserve from a more active cognitive reserve (Stern 2012). This concept of a potentially mobilizable brain reserve suggests that we have the ability to confront changes in the brain that occur due to age or pathological conditions even when they show no clinical symptoms or signs. Fundamental research has shown the role of a certain number of factors, including education, stress management, physical activity, sleep, social network, and leisure activities, in delaying the onset of Alzheimer's symptoms (see, for example, Barnes and Yaffe 2011). Pursuit of this set of disciplines in adulthood could allow us to maintain our cognitive and intellectual abilities as we age.

Brain Training

On the cognitive plane, brain training exercises strengthen the capacities of working memory. On the cellular plane, they increase synaptic and dendritic tree formation.

The software industry that offers products for exercising our memory and improving our cognitive abilities is now in full swing. But we can expand our horizons even further. Educational programs and video games are also worthwhile pursuits—on the condition that they further change and do not hamper you from spending time with other people. It is always better to play with other people than to play alone on your computer. No digital simulation can generate the emotional depths of direct human interaction.

Maintaining Social Networks

In the hippocampus, the integration of new memories depends upon the emotional content (not the rational content) of the experience. So while brain training exercises can promote neural plasticity, neurogenesis can take place in the hippocampus—the seat of Alzheimer's—only if the contents to be learned are permeated with emotion. Despite all the hype about using training software to stimulate our brain and keep our thinking sharp, it is simply not conceivable that dedicating time to computer exercises could, on its own, prevent or cure Alzheimer's disease. Our hunter-gatherer ancestors did not have these computer programs at their disposal. For brain training, they spent time with the members of their tribe, learning about each other and their history. It is most certainly in this ambiance of social networking that the hippocampus of a human being is best stimulated.

Physical Activity

The brain can be stimulated just as effectively by physical activity as it is by mental activity. It can be difficult to demonstrate the effectiveness of physical activity in isolation as a protective factor because the majority of physical activities also include both cognitive and social demands.

Those who devote themselves to physical activity are much less likely to develop Alzheimer's disease (or any form of dementia, for that matter), compared to people who are sedentary (Laurin et al. 2001). Even those who follow a light exercise program, such as simply taking a walk on a regular basis, have less risk of developing cognitive decline and Alzheimer's disease.

Physical activity has positive effects on our brain as a whole. Whether we are looking at our autobiographical memory or all our other cerebral faculties, all are improved by movement. This is how neurogenesis stimulated by physical exertion operates, leaving us better able to focus, to make good decisions, and to maintain our memory systems.

Performing adequate physical activity allows us to improve our cholesterol level, restore our cardiovascular system, and regulate our blood pressure. Furthermore, physical activity allows us to get better-quality sleep. All of these effects work together to reduce the risk of a hippocampic dementia (Alzheimer's) or a vascular incident (stroke).

The main goal should be to exercise regularly and to avoid the physical passivity that technological progress inspires. Thanks to this progress, our lives are more and more comfortable with respect to physical requirements, but now we can see that this is a poisoned gift.

In the context of the prevention or treatment of Alzheimer's disease, it is not necessary to practice high-level sports. It is easy to see that our hunter-gatherer ancestors had to move rather calmly, because if they had gone racing into the forest they would have scared away the game. In the same way, gathering fruits would have required them to take their time. Furthermore, hunter-gatherers would have kept moving for many hours (from four to six hours a day) to hunt and gather the food necessary for their survival.

Speak Several Languages

Studies have shown that bilingualism—which is to say, mastery of two languages—accelerates response to cognitive ability tests. Furthermore, Alzheimer's patients who speak several languages had a much less prominent degree of cerebral atrophy because of their larger cerebral reserve.

Get Good Sleep

As discussed in chapter 9, our brains are more active at night, when we are asleep, than when we are awake during the day. It is during deep sleep that new neurons are manufactured. Sleeping well is therefore vital to preserving our cognitive reserve and promoting neuroplasticity.

AWAKENING THE BRAIN IN ALZHEIMER'S PATIENTS

There are several ways to awaken the brain—that is, to tap in to the cognitive reserve and encourage neuroplasticity—in patients in the early stages of Alzheimer's.

Reminiscence

The most accessible method is to reminisce with patients, relying on old memories. Telling patients stories about their own lives is one way in which we can help bring other memories to the surface. This in turn will help them rediscover their identity in their own life story, building on the power of narrative identity.

Awaken the Emotions

The memories of the episodic memory banks are reinforced by emotion. Therefore, we can use photos, foods, aromas, films, and music to evoke memories, perhaps even memories of specific emotionally charged events. These evocations represent precious opportunities for people with Alzheimer's to express themselves, to tell stories, sing, move around, and imitate the gestures specific to a job, a sport, or dance.

Physical contact, too, offers an additional, sometimes indescribable effect in evoking memories.

Stimulate the Senses

The senses provide direct access to neural networks, and our sense memories—memories associated with certain sounds, sights, smells, tastes—are powerful triggers for emotional responses, activating the hippocampus.

When exploring the senses with Alzheimer's patients, the element of play should prevail over all other considerations. We can, for example, play music, especially recordings from patients' younger years, and encourage them to sing. Singing with them is essential, as it allows us to share the same joys. This sort of musical therapy is based on the nonverbal qualities and emotional power of the music. This active musical expression makes it possible to restore a certain sense of harmony in the patient by means of singing, playing a musical instrument, or listening to a specific song.

The Snoezelen method uses stimulation of all five senses at once. In a room that has been set up for this purpose, the patient's sight, hearing, touch, taste, and smell are stimulated.

THE THREE MAJOR PERIODS
OF BRAIN DEVELOPMENT

1. In Utero

The brain is constantly being reshaped and reorganized, and its plasticity assumes a constant interplay between construction and disintegration. This process, which neurobiologist Jean-Pierre Changeux describes as the "epigenesis of neuronal networks by selective stabilization of synapses" (Changeux et al. 1973), reaches its height during earliest infancy. Starting around the eighteenth week of pregnancy, the bulk of our one hundred billion neurons (a large number of which are doomed to die, mainly during the fetal period) are constructed and have found their way to their intended destinations.

Philippe Lambert (2006) tells us:

The liaisons between them—the synaptic connections—proliferate exuberantly. Under the influence of the infant's in utero experiences and during its first years of life, a number of them that are either redundant or irrelevant are going to be eliminated, while others will be consolidated. The end of these critical phases of development obviously doesn't spell the end of cerebral plasticity, but it will reduce the intensity of its manifestations. The child has to learn everything (walking, talking . . .), whereas the adult already enjoys many achievements.

In a certain way, plasticity is under the command of the environment. Studies have shown how important the intrauterine environment (yes, even then) is for good brain development. For example, children born of an undernourished mother will possess fewer neurons than children born of a well-nourished mother, and this will have an effect on their intellectual capacities.

2. Development

Functioning networks of neurons are established. This maturation is achieved through a precise program. The repercussion of all environmental factors is decisive.

Furthermore, the availability of nutrients (omega-3s and antioxidants) ensures cellular membrane fluidity.

The so-called adult stage of the brain is characterized by a certain stability in the neuronal structures.

3. Cerebral Aging

This stage marks the end of the stability that characterizes the previous stage. This stage, which lasts a long time, will be largely influenced by the surrounding environment. On the one hand, this can be a period of neuronal decay and death and the loss of dendritic and synaptic structures, and on the other, it can be a time of renewed creation characterized by maintained dendritic growth and expanded synapses.

The brain's plasticity is what permits us in large measure to maintain the effectiveness of the neural network of connections and our mental functions. So should we take back Santiago Ramón y Cajal's Nobel Prize because he proclaimed that neurogenesis was completely absent following birth? Luckily for us, he was completely wrong! For this reason it is possible for a protocol for preventing Alzheimer's disease to be initiated.

This undertaking should be primarily preventive, meaning before the disease has established itself or been identified. And it should also be used preventively secondarily for patients in whom this disease has been diagnosed. In this way, we can mobilize the remaining brain capacity and push back as far as possible the transition to the stages where pronounced dementia and loss of autonomy have become irreversible.

WHEN OUR BRAIN
THWARTS CHRONOS (TIME)

Are we really condemned to see our life expectancy continue to rise, thanks to the progress made by medical science, while our mental faculties continue to deteriorate during the last years of life? As we've seen in this chapter, that scenario is not inevitable. Certain regions of our brain, though admitedly limited in scope, possess the ability to renew their neurons at any age. From birth to death, our brain is constantly reorganizing itself, both by creating new neural connections and by creating new neurons, to adjust to the incessant changes of our environment.

This neuroplasticity, as it is called, depends little on our genetic inheritance but mainly on our life experiences. The richer our life experiences, the greater our neuroplasticity.

Perhaps most interestingly, in terms of preventing and treating Alzheimer's disease, the two cerebral structures we have identified as being capable of neurogenesis are the hippocampus and the olfactory bulb. As Professor Pierre-Marie Lledo (2019), head of the memory research unit at the Pasteur Institute, tells us:

> Like skin, liver, or blood, at least two mammalian brain structures are now known to be capable of permanently producing and receiving new neurons. These are the hippocampus, a key region for the formation of our memories and our affects, and the olfactory bulb, the first relay in the olfactory system that connects the sensory organ located in the nasal cavity to the cortex. . . .
>
> This research opens up unprecedented perspectives: an

astonishing range of possibilities for action and thoughts is available to us that could help us better adjust to the dynamics of the modern world, and also to intervene to repair our failing neural circuits, or to limit the decline in mental functions associated with age.

As Nietzsche said in *The Gay Science:* "Living—that is to continually eliminate from ourselves what is about to die."

BY WAY OF A CONCLUSION

We must laugh, sing, eat healthy foods, stimulate our sense of smell, maintain our social relations, have a blossoming sexuality, continue to learn, continue to draw on our neurons, and continue to exercise—at least 8,000 to 10,000 steps a day. Aging well must rhyme with pleasure!

Activity, intellectual stimulation, and interaction are therefore, with the quantity and quality of our sleep, the essential conditions to the formation of new neurons in the hippocampus, which gives us the arms we need to fight Alzheimer's. However, these new neurons can only develop and mature if we give our brain the food it needs. For our memory and cognitive skills to last into a ripe old age, the hippocampus requires three principal elements: building materials for the neurons in their developmental stage, energy, and protective agents.

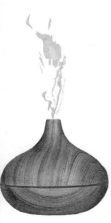

12

Alzheimer's Disease and the Sense of Smell

A Closer Look at Our Primary Sense

Taste and smell alone, more fragile but more enduring, more unsubstantial, more persistent, more faithful, remain poised a long time, like souls, remembering, waiting, hoping, amid the ruins of all the rest; and bear unflinchingly, in the tiny and almost impalpable drop of their essence, the vast structure of recollection.

MARCEL PROUST, *SWANN'S WAY*

THE MEMORY OF ODORS

Volatile aromatic molecules are captured by thousands of chemo-receptors in the olfactory epithelium and then transmitted to the center of the sense of smell, seated at the very heart of the limbic brain. There, every odor we perceive is compared with our obviously personal history of smells, where, based on information arising from our own memories and emotions, the odor will be classified as either pleasant or unpleasant, as attractive or repulsive. The obvious value of working with smell stems from the fact that it is the only one of our senses whose messages do not first travel through the neocortex. In a way that could be described as insidious (because it is unconscious), the active volatile agents go straight to the limbic brain and inspire a reaction independent of the will, which could permit the resolution of the behavioral issues found in Alzheimer's disease—namely, mood change, loss of motivation, apathy, anxiety, depression, intellectual decline, and agitation.

There is no cause for surprise in the fact that the sense of smell touches the deepest, most intimate part of the self. The power behind the throne and an infallible guide, the sense of smell is intimately connected to the greatest vital process for all living beings: breathing. Just as it is impossible to not breathe, it is equally delusional to try to not smell. This gives us a better understanding of sayings such as "something doesn't smell right," "comes out smelling like a rose," or "I smell a rat."

With its direct influence on our nervous system, smell is easily associated with intuition and, like it, initially affects us unconsciously. Smelling and feeling are simultaneous [and in French, the verb *sentir* can mean either —*Trans.*], and trusting what you feel, what a situation smells like, is a step more and more people are choosing to take.

The science that decodes the olfactory perceptions of the active principles of aromas is called aromachology, while the therapy that works with the neuro-olfactory receptors is called olfactotherapy.

Although olfactory problems are not in the primary clinical description of Alzheimer's disease, they are common and often overlooked both in clinical practice and in patients suffering from anosognosia, who are by and large unaware of their disorders. The literature of the past thirty years has shown evidence for early decline of the ability to smell in Alzheimer's disease, which becomes increasingly severe as the disease worsens.

In a 2010 issue of *La lettre du neurologue* [The Neurologist's Letter], S. Lombion, L. Rumbach, and J. L. Millot, of the neuroscience laboratory in Besançon, France, discussed their findings from studies on the relationship between the sense of smell and neurodegenerative diseases.

> Olfactory perception offers the originality of the initial and active combination of emotional components (hedonic aspects, pleasure, disagreeable, and so forth), and different kinds of cognitive processes (recognition, categorization, naming). Distinct neuronal networks are probably used to process these different operations. In comparison to other sensory stimulations, the emotional dimension of odors is particularly pervasive. Smells trigger emotional reactions of all kinds. They regulate our moods, give birth to intense experiences of pleasure or discomfort, feed our sympathies, and inspire soothing or jealous states. Implicitly or explicitly, they facilitate or hinder the course of thought.

These emotional influences are promptly transformed into choices, preferences, behaviors, and attractions or repulsions.

Like many other experts, the researchers established correspondences between alterations of the olfactory capacities and certain neurodegenerative diseases, which could result in a diagnostic tool and a way to foresee such illnesses.

THE SINGULAR FEATURES OF THE SENSE OF SMELL

The sense of smell distinguishes itself from the other sensory systems by several unique characteristics.

Neuroanatomical Circuitry

Because, over the course of human evolution, the olfactory system developed before that of the thalamus, the olfactory channels feed directly into the archaic structures located at the base of the brain. This is where the memory and emotional centers are located, with the limbic system, which mainly consists of the amygdala and the hippocampus. This means that the sense of smell has a privileged path of access to the brain. These singular features explain the highly emotional nature of odors and of olfactory memories. The processes in the base structures are automatic and unconscious, which is why, when we perceive an odor, our first reaction is emotional in nature and indicates whether we like it. It is only in the following phases that the olfactory connections expand toward the thalamus and the neocortex, while, in contrast, the other sensory systems are directly connected to the neocortex.

In fact, the olfactory system exhibits a singular anatomical organization because its neuroreceptors are directly connected to the amygdala and the hippocampus, in contrast to the sensory system of sight, whose paths cross through the neocortex before they reach the amygdala. There is thus a privileged anatomical connection between smell, emotion, and memory.

Embryogenesis

In addition to its unique circuitry, the sensory organs associated with the sense of smell are the first to form during embryogenesis. As Schaal et al. (2004) tell us, "from the end of the first gestational trimester, the main olfactory system has receptor neurons that look morphologically mature" and fetal olfaction becomes functional in the twenty-ninth week of gestation. The first olfactory experiences occur in utero. Schaal et al. conclude that "olfaction mediates a thread of sensory continuity between the prenatal and postnatal environments."

THE PRIMARY ANATOMICAL STRUCTURES INVOLVED IN SMELL

The olfactory system consists of three subsystems:

+ The general, or primary, system. Stimulation of this system causes a sensation of smell, prompting a conscious behavior.
+ The trigeminal system. Stimulation of this system causes a somatic sensory sensation (a tactile sensation, or a sensation of heat, pain, or moistness).
+ The vomeronasal system. This system detects pheromones and prompts unconscious behavior of a sexual overtone.

In human beings, although less developed, the vomeronasal organ, also known as Jacobson's organ, is located as a paired structure at the base of the nasal septum. It is functionally and anatomically distinct from the primary olfactory system. If this organ is destroyed in an animal, it will lose all appetite for sex!

Olfactory Neurons

Olfactory neurons, representing 60 to 80 percent of nerve receptor cells, capture odors and transmit information about them. Their axons allow the conduction of nerve impulses carrying that information into the olfactory bulb. All the olfactory neurons together form the olfactory nerve.

Support Cells

Support cells protect the olfactory neurons by different means:

+ They break down foreign organic molecules present in the nasal cavity.

✦ They isolate the olfactory neurons from one another.

✦ They produce potassium ions (K+), which are important for creating active electrical potential and transmitting information.

The Olfactory Bulb

The olfactory neurons eventually merge together and form the olfactory bulb, which is located at the anterior end of the encephalon. Its role is to process the olfactory information brought by the olfactory neurons. In fact, it processes and encodes this information before sending it toward the higher structures of the brain. The olfactory bulb's purpose is to shape the message to be as clear and specific as possible.

The Brain

The olfactory bulb passes information to the encephalon by three paths:

✦ The lateral tractus (lateral path). This path leads from the olfactory bulb to the primary olfactory cortex. Then the afferent information is sent toward the thalamus and the limbic system (hippocampus and amygdala), which are responsible for processing emotions, hence the emotional associations that are often strongly tied to certain odors.

✦ The middle tractus (middle path). This path leads from the olfactory bulb to the olfactory tubercule (an extension of the olfactory bulb) and then to the thalamus.

✦ The median tractus (the median path). This path leads from the olfactory bulb to the orbitalfrontal cortex and then the thalamus.

DISORDERS OF THE OLFACTORY SYSTEM

Disorders of the sense of smell are often called dysosmia. Loss of the sense of smell is often called anosmia. Anosmia is often accompanied by a set of varied problems, including a period of severe depression.

The specific attack against the olfactory system in Alzheimer's disease, combined with its connection with the limbic structures and the strong emotional power of the olfactory memory, form a good argument in favor of the clinical value of studying olfactory disorders in this disease.

Olfactory disorders are not specific to Alzheimer's. They are also present in other neurodegenerative diseases, like Parkinson's disease, Lewy body disease, vascular dementia, and frontotemporal dementia, and in certain psychiatric disorders like schizophrenia or depression. The processes that are altered differ between Alzheimer's and Parkinson's but are sometimes similar in other neurodegenerative diseases. So studies of olfactory disorders may hold great value in a differential diagnosis. These diagnostic implications are essential for the improvement and prevention of the therapy (Sohrabi et al. 2012).

The Quantitative Disturbances

Anosmia

Loss of the sense of smell can include all smells or only some of them (specific anosmia). It is often coupled with dysgeusia (loss of taste). However, this loss of the sense of smell can be due to blockages in the sinuses—namely, nasal polyps (related to allergies).

Hyposmia

This is a more moderate reduction of the ability to smell, which is often due to trauma or chronic infections. It can also be of genetic or congenital origin.

Hyperosmia

In hyperosmia, olfactory capacity is visibly intensified. This symptom can be seen in people afflicted with cluster headaches, migraines, or chronic adrenocortical insufficiency.

Qualitative Disorders

Cacosmia

Patients with cacosmia smell fetid, putrid odors or other things they find disagreeable. This particular disorder can have a physiological origin (rhinitis, sinusitis, tumor) or a psychological origin.

Ozena, a chronic disease of the nose that bears some resemblance, is a form of rhinitis characterized by a foul-smelling discharge.

Parosmia

This condition is an inability to correctly identify odors. Instead, odors are misinterpreted as the smell of rot, excrement, or chemicals.

Phantosmia

This condition involves the perception of "ghost" odors. The smells can be pleasant or unpleasant.

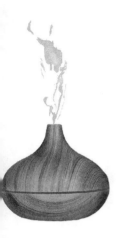

13

Finding Help from Essential Oils

The Benefits and Practice of Olfactory Therapy

BECAUSE ALZHEIMER'S disease is incurable, the relief offered by nonpharmaceutical intervention has become an important strategy for management of the condition.

We know that the olfactory system is the sense organ that is closest to the brain. Knowing also that the sense of smell's central system animates zones that have been damaged in Alzheimer's patients, we can see that stimulation of this sense, or olfactory therapy, can form an effective nonpharmaceutical treatment.

Olfactory therapy can have a wide range of effects:

+ Creating a sense of well-being
+ Developing acquired memories of odors
+ Creating or re-creating temporal-spatial references
+ Creating olfactory anchor points
+ Encouraging identity reconstruction through the use of referential odors

Essential Oils Prescribed at Hospitals

Slowly and discreetly, but surely, aromatherapy is becoming established in a growing number of hospitals in the United States and Europe. From a simply relaxing diffusion to genuine therapeutic application, its use is becoming more accepted professionally, and its use as a more natural yet effective treatment for the greater benefit of patients, families, and caregivers is transforming the medical world.

Even just a few years ago, the few nurses and doctors using aromatherapy in a hospital setting preferred to keep silent about the practice, given the medical establishment's reluctance to embrace alternative treatments. However, little by little, under growing pressure from the public, with support provided by scientific studies and conclusive experiments, more hospitals around the world have become receptive, and more and more of them have given their blessing to the use of essential oils within their white walls.

Geriatric and palliative care departments were among the first to take an interest in aromatherapy. Elderly patients often take a variety of medications and are more sensitive to the side effects of established treatments, inspiring these medical bodies to look for ways to integrate other forms of care. A number of nursing homes have also begun to use essential oils.

THE MULTIPLE EFFECTS OF ESSENTIAL OILS

Aromatherapy has naturally expanded the palette of treatments available to therapists. Rigorous protocols have been established (including medical prescription, traceability, and testing), and caregivers have become trained in aromatherapy and the use of essential oils so they can successfully integrate them into their existing practices.

For example, a combination of wintergreen and katafray essential oils diluted with vegetable oil offers quick relief for joint pain, thereby allowing the use of powerful analgesics to be limited.

To calm the frequent anxiety, anguish, and agitation of Alzheimer's patients, some hospitals turn to the essential oils of lavender, sweet orange, and chamomile as inhalants (either from an oil-soaked handkerchief or an individual smell stick) and as ointments on the back, the arch of the foot, the sternum, or the inner wrists.

Melissa is the essential oil that is most widely used for helping patients at the end of their life let go. This type of management for end-of-life care provides substantial improvement to helping patients and their loved ones. It puts the emphasis on the "care" in caregivers.

In addition to their therapeutic properties, essential oils can help reawaken the mind in Alzheimer's patients. The direct connection of the sense of smell with the cerebral structures that govern emotions and memory make it possible to use scent to elicit emotionally charged memories—reminscences, so to speak. These little bits of autobiographical detail can restore to patients a piece of themselves, of their identity, and can help combat the apathy and depression that often accompany Alzheimer's.

WHICH ESSENTIAL OILS TO CHOOSE

We have a wide range of essential oils from which to choose for stimulating our olfactory system and challenging the symptoms of Alzheimer's.

Cerebral Stimulants

Rosemary essential oil is a memory stimulant and promotes attention and alertness as well. It allows for improved quality of life for individuals suffering from dementia by helping with both memory and mood.

The essential oils of peppermint, ginger, and cypress also exhibit stimulating properties, and their tonic qualities support cognitive function.

Lavender and lavandin both have high levels of linalool, a monoterpene alcohol, and can improve the ability to memorize.

Monoterpenes can also be found in the essential oils of members of the citrus family (lemon, orange, mandarin orange) and the conifers (balsam fir, black spruce, Scotch pine). These essential oils function as cortico-adrenal stimulants and analgesics, and their stimulating effect makes it possible to maintain mental activity and a certain level of alertness.

Marjoram

Marjoram is traditionally known for its calming properties, but it is also a tonic. Nervous patients going through a decompensation phase, who are not sleeping, have lost weight, and are feeling restless and fearful, will benefit greatly from the 4-terpineol (and other alcohols and monoterpenes) contained in the essential oil, which will allow them to recharge their psycho-neuro-endocrine-immune axis. Once they have been fully recharged this way, the patients will feel a true, deep sense of calm, not the counterfeit provided by antidepressant pharmaceuticals and sleeping pills.

Neroli

Neroli (the flowers of bitter orange) essential oil is indispensable in neurology. It is antidepressive, combats high blood pressure, rebalances the mental-emotional sphere, reduces stress, calms agitation, and facilitates falling sleep. By its action on the central nervous system, it regulates anxieties, sorrow, and tears.

Lavender

Quite often, patients are stressed and spasmodic. Before any treatment, I recommend that they be helped to relax, and for this, we can use lavender essential oil. It contains two active principles: linalool and linalyl acetate. It is a powerful antispasmodic, it is calming and relaxing, and it lowers blood pressure. It targets the same regions of the brain as pharmaceutical antidepressants, and it is indicated for stress, worry, anxiety, and trouble sleeping.

Its absorption into the bloodstream by way of the respiratory tract is the source of direct effects on the brain cell receptors, such as the receptors of gamma-aminobutyric acid (GABA), a neurotransmitter that helps with regulating things such as appetite, sleep, and memory.

Essential Oils to Restore Acetylcholine

Among the numerous anomalies affecting neurotransmitters in Alzheimer's disease, it is currently possible to take action on two of them: the deficiency in acetylcholine and the excess of glutamate (on N-methyl-D-aspartate, or NMDA, receptors).

Acetylcholine plays a role in the brain's cognitive function and in mood regulation. To increase the available quantity of acetylcholine, physicians often prescribe anticholinesterase drugs, which block the natural breakdown of acetylcholine. The same inhibitory effect can be achieved by the use of certain essential oils, without the side effects inherent in pharmaceutical treatments. Certain molecules in these essential oils bind to the anticholinesterase enzyme, thereby inhibiting its breakdown of acetylcholine in the brain.

One essential oil often used for this purpose is rosemary (*Rosmarinus officinalis*), which contains high levels of monoterpenes, especially 1,8-cineole. Rosemary's inhibitory effect on acetylcholinesterase is thought to be due to the synergistic effect of 1,8-cineole and another of rosemary's constituents, alpha-pinene.

Other essential oils with high levels of monoterpenes, like *Eucalyptus globulus,* have similar inhibitory effects on the acetylcholinesterase enzyme.

Neurorestorative Essential Oils of Madagascar

When I was working in the city of Antsirabe, in Madagascar, teaching aromatherapy to fifty doctors and treating five hundred orphans, I took advantage of my time to study the essential oils native to the island. I focused on the essential oils that can treat neurodegenerative and mental diseases, and I was able to expand my knowledge about aromatherapy thanks to the valuable advice of Simon Lemesle, the head of a company that produces and promotes Madagascar's essential oils.

The quality of the fragrances, the therapeutic effectiveness, the tolerance, and the delicacy of their effect on the psyche are entirely connected to the balance and vitality of the specific essential oil being used. Not all the essential oils of katafray, for example, have as profound an effect on inflammation and emotions, nor do all the essential oils of saro procure such a remarkable galvanizing and protective effect.

Butterfly Ginger Essential Oil

This essential oil, obtained from the leaves of butterfly ginger, has a very balanced effect on the nervous system. Butterfly ginger provides remarkable support to individuals who are prone to depression and have little trust in themselves. Strengthening, motivating, and promoting expression of our personality, it can be used every morning by applying one or two drops on the wrists.

A protective essential oil that combats stress, it is helpful to people who are too wrapped up in everyday life and in material things. Used in massage or olfactory therapy, butterfly ginger leads to a deep feeling of inner peace but also pushes us to connect with the outside world. Its liberating effect remains contained within the earthly principle of the plants of the Zingiberaceae family.

Lacking any aggressive properties, it is easily tolerated by the skin and can be applied undiluted to the inside of the wrists or diluted in plant oil for massage along the spinal column. Or it can simply be used for inhalation. Its production by distillation is small, so this remains a rare, precious, and intriguing essential oil.

Grains of Paradise Essential Oil

Fruity and sweet, the fragrance of grains of paradise essential oil has nothing comparable to it in aromatherapy. Its fragrance seems to envelop us and enter us with great gentleness. The essential oil pulls us together, allowing us to come back to ourselves and perform inner work.

When used in the evening, the essential oil promotes sleepiness and bodes well for a good night's sleep. It also softens dreams and diminishes nightmares. A very small amount inhaled or applied to the skin is adequate; open the vial, breathe calmly and deeply several times, then apply one drop on the inner surface of one wrist and massage it with the other wrist.

The essential oil for cocooning, grains of paradise is a refined treatment for getting back in touch with yourself after a day's work or after a period of feeling overwhelmed or depressed.

The essential oil of butterfly ginger seems to be the perfect complement for grains of paradise. Preferably the ginger would be used during the morning and at the start of treatment, and the grains of paradise during the evening and on your days off.

Herbe des Rois Essential Oil

The incredibly intense fragrance of "herb of kings" essential oil has an overwhelmingly positive effect on the mind. Its immediate rebalancing effect on the nervous system creates a profound sense of relaxation and a sovereign state of mellowness, followed by a unique sense of detachment that brings with it improved attention and perception.

Recently its applications have been expanded to treatment of nervous system disorders such as the neurological consequences of Lyme disease.

Even just simple contact with this plant during its harvesting, and even more so during its distillation, can yield its powerfully purifying and uplifting properties. These experiences, as well as observation of the plant and its winged stems, reveal a perfectly structured union of the elements of earth and air. This is likely the most splendid revelation of Madagascan flora.

Katafray Essential Oil

The discreet fragrance of katafray essential oil offers a sweet woody note that is amazingly luminous, enveloping and soothing us like a balm that has come to relieve all suffering. An excellent broad and multivalent anti-inflammatory, it is a primary essential oil for the locomotor (or musculoskeletal) system: muscles, joints, and tendons. It also figures prominently in the formulation of massage oils and can be applied over a painful area for relief. An essential oil of movement, it rebalances the adrenal glands without excessively invigorating them and helps recharge our batteries during periods of convalescence or burnout. Applying it to the lower back every morning will bring courage and determination; it can help us remain firm and not go off course while taking the drama out of everyday situations. It conveys a sense of being anchored, which is good for restorative sleep.

If you take the time to explore this essential oil, through olfactory therapy, for example, you will witness an extremely penetrating effect on the mind through the awakening of ancestral impressions and emotions.

Manavao Essential Oil

In Malagasy, *manavao* means "renewal." This essential oil provides an intense sense of recentering. By freeing the emotions, manavao brings a deep sense of relaxation that is exhibited physically by a loosening of the muscles and a moderation of the heartbeat. Emotions become calm, gentle, and balanced.

The quantity of essential oil obtained through distillation is quite low, but it is extremely potent. Those who know its virtues use it to improve cognitive abilities, perception, and intuition. It is indicated for emotional shocks, heartbreak, and professional burnout, as well as situations in which we are having difficulty finding our footing.

For olfactory therapy, manavao can be rubbed lightly onto the wrists, behind the ears, or even on the solar plexus. Diluted in plant oil, it is also excellent for massage.

Saro Essential Oil

In a society where psychic and physical attacks are inevitable, saro offers peerless protection. With its great vital energy, saro can be compared to a veritable suit of armor or the rampart of a castle.

Applying or simply smelling saro essential oil can be an intense experience. It is at first invigorating; its fresh and slightly acidic fragrance powerfully but not aggressively penetrates the entire respiratory tract. Following this, a sensation of relaxation can be felt, coupled with a sense of thinking clearly and lucidly. A feeling of harmony and openness settles in, which guides us to a state of unique awareness.

Applying saro on the wrists every morning will awaken, motivate, and protect. You will feel courageous, protected by this fragrance, as if all your problems and difficulties have simply vanished, leaving you feeling purified, as if a poison has been removed from your body.

TREATING ALZHEIMER'S WITH ESSENTIAL OILS

For patients afflicted with Alzheimer's, I recommend a two-part treatment with essential oils:

- ✦ Stimulating essential oils in the morning (black spruce, sea pine, woodrose, ylang-ylang, and so on)
- ✦ Calming essential oils in the evening (bergamot, frankincense, lavender, neroli, marjoram, and so on)

You can try one or two essential oils at a time, or you can use one of the synergistic blends described below. Put twenty drops into an atomizer (an ultrasound diffuser) and run it in the patient's room for about twenty minutes.

A Morning Blend

Synergy for Stimulating Alertness and Memory

30% rosemary (chemotype cineole) essential oil

20% black spruce essential oil

20% lavender essential oil

20% lemon essential oil

10% garden marjoram essential oil

Evening Blends

You will find three possible blends here. These synergies make it possible to calm a patient and restore a certain level of harmony; all reduce stress levels and allow for a better quality of sleep. It is important to identify which one works best for the patient in order to suggest its regular diffusion in their room.

Synergy No. 1

Chamomile essential oil

Lemon verbena essential oil

Neroli essential oil

Synergy No. 2

Lavandin essential oil

Saro essential oil

Ylang-ylang essential oil

Synergy No. 3

Lavender essential oil

Neroli essential oil

Sandalwood essential oil

Formulas Using Neroli (Bitter Orange Flower)

For Melancholy or Mild Depression

Rosewood essential oil	2 ml
Bergamot essential oil	1 ml
Garden marjoram essential oil	1 ml
Neroli essential oil	0.5 ml
Apricot kernel oil	5.5 ml

Dosage: Three or four drops on the solar plexus or on the inside of the wrists, repeated as often as needed.

For Severe Insomnia

Chamomile essential oil	2 ml
Neroli essential oil	1 ml
Ylang-ylang essential oil	0.5 ml
Apricot kernel oil	6 ml

Dosage: Four drops on the arch of each foot, on the solar plexus, and on the inside of the wrists, at bedtime.

For End-of-Life Distress or Hyperexcitability

Frankincense essential oil	1 ml
Angelica root essential oil	0.5 ml
Neroli essential oil	0.5 ml
Apricot kernel oil	8 ml

Dosage: Four drops on the arch of each foot, on the solar plexus, and on the inside of the wrists, at bedtime.

METHODS OF APPLICATION

Inhalation

Inhalation through the nasal passages is recommended for treating nervous system disorders (stress, emotions, behaviors) and neurological disorders (Alzheimer's, Parkinson's, and so on) using essential oil–based olfactory therapy. The purpose is to exploit the informational activity of every essential oil fragrance that has a connection with the patient's life experience so as to regulate and balance all psycho-emotional reactions.

Breathing in the aroma of the essential oil directly from the bottle, or from a tissue on which you've placed several drops of essential oil, is the easiest method. Making this a habit two or three times a day, for a period of one to two minutes, should suffice. The simplicity of this method makes it possible to easily use a group of essential oils, choosing from among them in response to individual symptoms.

You could also practice a small ritual of putting several drops of diluted essential oil on the inside of your wrists, then cupping your hands over your nose and taking a long, deep breath. Repeat three times in succession. You can do this as often as you like.

Diffusion

Diffusion of essential oils in the air is helpful for

- ✦ cleansing the air, essentially biologically purifying it; and
- ✦ managing behavioral issues and mood in neurodegenerative diseases.

Air Diffusers

There are two kinds of devices for diffusing essential oils in the air: ultrasonic diffusers and nebulizing diffusers. The latter uses an electric pump to atomize the aromatic volatile molecules and spray them into the air, while the ultrasonic diffuser uses water. The nebulizer allows a greater concentration of essential oils in the air. It is better for larger public spaces and areas where people congregate: waiting rooms, businesses, retirement homes, nursing homes, and hospitals. Diffusing antimicrobial essential oils in these sorts of group spaces can offer people greater immunity against infections.

Ultrasonic diffusion is more suitable for home use. Because it diffuses essential oils into the air while also humidifying the air, it is less concentrated in a smaller space, and people are better able to tolerate the essential oils.

Essential Oils for Diffusing

Not all essential oils are suitable for diffusing. Some should *not* be diffused, such as essential oils with high levels of phenols (savory, clove, thyme, rock rose, wintergreen, helichrysum, marjoram, niaouli, mountain savory, tea tree), which are irritating for the respiratory mucous membranes, and essential oils with ketones (see the warning below).

Warning: Neurotoxicity

In neurological diseases such as Parkinson's, Alzheimer's, convulsions, epilepsy, and so forth, it is extremely important to avoid essential oils that have high levels of terpene ketones.

In small doses, ketones stimulate the nervous system and can cause sympathicotonia. In high doses, they are neurotoxins and stupefying.

The excited or stimulated state that is first visible is followed by neurotoxic disturbances, such as nausea, vomiting, dizziness, trouble talking, and mental confusion, then stupefaction, then depression, and finally coma. The nerve toxicity of these molecules depends on a variety of criteria that, in descending order of importance, include the dose administered, the ketone molecule, the concentration of the molecule in the essential oil, the way it is administered, and the duration of the treatment.

Ketones can be recognized by their biochemical structure as indicated by a name ending with -one (verbenone, menthone, borneone, thujone, piperitone, crypton, and so forth). They are found in the following essential oils:

- Caraway
- Eucalyptus (E. globulus)
- Fennel
- Helichrysum
- Pennyroyal
- Peppermint
- Rosemary chemotype verbenone
- Sage
- Spearmint

The following essential oils are well suited to diffusion and can be helpful in treatments for Alzheimer's patients:

Balsam fir
Bergamot (calming)
Bitter orange
Black pepper (digestive tonic)
Black spruce (general tonic)
Cajeput (expectorant)
Citron (stomachic)
Eastern hemlock (restores nervous system balance)
Eucalyptus radiata
Eucalyptus smithii (antiviral)
Field mint
Frankincense (antidepressant)
Goldenrod (anti-inflammatory)
Grapefruit (atmospheric antiseptic)
Green myrtle
Inula (mucolytic when diffused)
Japanese cedar (analgesic)
Java citronella
Larch (nerve tonic)
Lavandin
Lavender (in combination)
Lemon (purgative)
Lemon eucalyptus (anti-inflammatory)
Lemon verbena (sedative)
Lemongrass
Mandarin (relaxing)
Manuka (antihistamine)
Neroli (restores balance to the nervous system)

Orange

Palmarosa

Peppermint (in small quantities)

Ravintsara (immune stimulant)

Red myrtle (for unclogging arteries)

Rhododendron (relaxing)

Rosemary chemotype cineole

Rosewood (for neurasthenia)

Sandalwood (urinary and pulmonary antiseptic)

Scented geranium

Scotch pine (nerve and sex tonic)

Siberian fir (respiratory antiseptic)

Tea tree (anti-infectious)

Vanilla (hydrates skin)

Verbena (powerful sedative)

Ylang-ylang (anti-anxiety)

Massage

Touching a body is an act of reconciliation with a human being. Touching the skin means touching the brain. In embryology, the ectoderm is the first of the three primary germ layers—that is, groups of cells—to emerge, and eventually it differentiates into two structures: the skin and the brain. In other words, the skin and brain are twin organs, giving off the same vibration.

The skin and its mucous membranes offer a significant path for safe applications of treatment for a number of disorders. Considering that drops of essential oil represent little biochemical bombs, a few drops will suffice.

For older children and adults, the customary dose will range from eight to fifteen drops per application. This dose can be applied neat, without being diluted, as long as it is not one that is caustic or irritating. Nevertheless, dilution with a plant oil (in a 50:50 ratio) is recommended for the first treatments, and in most cases, dilution is called for.

The best oils for this purpose are apricot kernel, macadamia, sea buckthorn, sesame, sweet almond, and tamanu (from *Calophyllum* species).

The following massage oil formulations can be of benefit for patients with Alzheimer's.

For Phobias, Nightmares, or Obsessions

Angelica root essential oil	1 ml
Apricot kernel oil	9 ml

Use this formula in the evening, or three or four times a day depending on the severity of the symptoms. Apply four drops on the arch of each foot, on the solar plexus, and on the inside of the wrists.

For Extrasystoles, Palpitations, or Irritability

Chamomile essential oil	1 ml
Frankincense essential oil	1 ml
Angelica root essential oil	0.5 ml
Apricot kernel oil	7.5 ml

Apply four drops on the solar plexus and/or in the mouth with a little honey or cane sugar. Or apply four drops on the arch of each foot, on the solar plexus, and on the inside of the wrists, at bedtime.

For Worry, Anxiety, or Insomnia

Yuzu essential oil	1 ml
Angelica root essential oil	0.5 ml
Lavender essential oil	0.5 ml
Marjoram essential oil	0.5 ml
Apricot kernel oil	7.5 ml

Apply four drops on the solar plexus and/or in the mouth with a little honey or cane sugar. Or apply four drops on the arch of each foot, on the solar plexus, and on the inside of the wrists, at bedtime.

For Agitation or Excitation

Petitgrain essential oil	2 ml
Yuzu essential oil	1 ml
Neroli essential oil	0.5 ml
Apricot kernel oil	6.5 ml

Apply four drops on the solar plexus, in the mouth, and/or on the inside surface of the wrists. Repeat as needed.

SYNERGISTIC BLENDS FOR SYSTEMATIC BALANCE

These synergistic blends work to introduce a balancing effect into your daily life.

Air Synergy

*Attain bodily peace and mental tranquillity,
and meditate in the boundless freedom of the sky for
every day to be a good day.*

This synergy is recommended for feeling uplifted, meditating, clearing your mind, creating, and imagining. It is associated with the air element, the color white, and springtime.

> 15 drops *Helichrysum gymnocephalum* essential oil
>
> 5 drops *Croton geayi* essential oil
>
> 3 drops rosemary chemotype verbenone essential oil
>
> 2 drops Bourbon geranium essential oil

Water Synergy

*Like a stream of pure water flowing over a gentle slope,
let go of your daily stress and anxiety and return to
the fullness of a high mountain lake.*

This synergy is recommended for removing stress, purification, and distancing yourself from difficulties. It is ideal taken in the evening as a relaxant. It is associated with the water element, the color blue, and winter.

> 9 drops lemon eucalyptus essential oil
>
> 8 drops niaouli essential oil
>
> 8 drops ylang-ylang extra essential oil

Earth Synergy

*Draw from the heart of the Earth's generous energy for
its original strength and vitality.*

This synergy is used for motivation, boosting morale, acceptance, revitalization, and making a decision. It is associated with the earth element, the color chestnut brown, and autumn.

> 8 drops katafray essential oil
> 7 drops iary (arina) essential oil
> 6 drops *Helichrysum bracteiferum* essential oil
> 4 drops saro essential oil

Fire Synergy

*Warm and sensual for those who know how to control it, fire will
warm the body and the heart but, like love, will burn the unwary.*

This synergy is intended to foster better communication, sharing, and love. It is associated with the fire element, the color red, and summer.

> 14 drops ylang-ylang complete essential oil
> 10 drops saro essential oil
> 1 drop (or less) cinnamon essential oil

First Forest Synergy

An unforgettable olfactory journey—then a
return to the source of energy.

This invigorating synergy restores balance to the nervous system. It can be applied daily to the wrists and lower back. It can also be diffused.

11 drops katafray essential oil

11 drops saro essential oil

3 drops butterfly ginger essential oil

Eubiotic Synergy

This blend has invigorating, stimulating, and protective properties that bring about a complete and lasting revitalization of the body. It should be used from the beginning of winter, during times of epidemics, or when you are feeling a loss of tone.

18 drops saro essential oil

3 drops palmarosa essential oil

3 drops rosemary chemotype verbenone essential oil

1 drop (or less) cinnamon essential oil

The proportions provided above will make 1 ml (twenty-five drops) of synergy that can be used undiluted on the wrists or another spot on the skin. First test for tolerance, which you can do by dabbing a little in the fold of the elbow, especially for the blends containing cinnamon essential oil. If your skin is reactive, combine the 1 ml of essential oil blend with 9 ml of plant-based oil (almond, hazelnut, and tamanu oils are good choices) to make a massage oil that is just 10 percent essential oil. These synergy blends can also be used simply for inhalation or in diffusers, and the eubiotic synergy can also be taken orally.

To end the chapter, I would like to cite the edifying testimony of Nelly Rabeau, a caregiver for elderly and Alzheimer's patients at Saint-Nicolas Hospital in Angers, France, who was interviewed by journalist Sophie Bartczak in 2015.

> Since aromatherapy was introduced in 2010, my profession has taken on a whole new dimension. Essential oils are now part of my daily life and bring a lot to me personally. Before a relaxing session of touch therapy, I set up the diffuser, which allows me to refocus and be in a better listening position. I am no longer just "doing" but am in a relationship with the other person, and this changes everything. The combination of touch and essential oils is an extraordinary vector of relationship. It goes beyond words, age, disease. It allows very intense relationships to form, with confidences shared and, sometimes, even tears. Once when I was giving a foot massage to a woman in her nineties, who hadn't spoken for several years, she blurted out, "She is good, Janine," speaking of herself. A beautiful moment etched in my memory. Aromatherapy transformed my job.

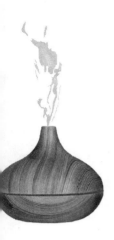

14

The Cooking
of Food

Problems and Solutions

AS MENTIONED in chapter 1, our ancestors went through two major dietary phases: that of the raw, which was ruled by the sense of smell, and that of the cooked, which was dominated by the sense of taste. Millennia ago, our ancestors relied on the olfactory system as their primary warning against danger. But as paleoanthropologists have discovered, over the course of time, facing repeated aggression from foreign molecules introduced mainly by high-temperature cooking, the olfactory system underwent significant genetic mutations that led to the erosion of our primitive survival and adaptation instinct.

Cooking foods at high temperatures alters the structure of certain molecules, causing them to become new compounds that our cells and enzymes do not recognize. These molecular transformations (combined with the destruction of many vitamins, such as B_3, B_6, B_9, and B_{12}) cause changes not only in the appearance of the food but also in its taste, its tenderness (which makes it easier to consume meat), and most importantly its digestibility.

This is why some vegetables that are tasteless or bitter when raw, and sometimes indigestible or with a repulsive odor (a signal of potential toxicity, as is the case for potatoes, manioc, green beans, and grains), are able to be eaten without any apparent harm when they are cooked, with the ultimate concern now being only the search for gustatory pleasure!

OVERWHELMING THE METABOLISM

The everyday culinary art of cooking with heat, which appears entirely banal, is not inconsequential. Under elevated heat levels, all methods—steaming, pressure-cooking, baking, blanching, grilling, broiling, and boiling, not to mention by microwaving, which has its own specific and variable consequences—cause the molecules in food to collide, break, and cling randomly to other structures to form new, extremely complex combinations that do not exist in nature.

A sugar molecule and a protein molecule, when combined under heat, undergo the Maillard reaction, creating molecules that are not physiologically able to be assimilated by the human body. They cannot be metabolized and consequently engender dysbiosis (disruption of the intestinal microbiome and intestinal permeability). With cooking, sugars polymerize and oils oxidize and cyclize. Isomers can form, and while our digestive system is filled with enzymes to help us break down food, those enzymes are programmed to act only on the original natural substances, not isomers, and so we are unable to metabolize them either.

The longer food is cooked and the higher the temperature, the more significant the destruction of catalysts and nutrients will be, for example:

Over 122°F: destruction of some enzymes
Over 140°F: destruction of vitamin C
Over 194°F: destruction of some B vitamins and vitamin E
Over 212°F: precipitation of mineral salts and trace elements into indigestible flakes; oxidation of fat-soluble vitamins A and D

Over 248°F: destruction of the remaining vitamins (B₂, B₃, E); breakdown of lipids into tars and benzopyrene (smoke from oils)

LEUKOCYTOSIS

In the 1930s, at the Institute of Clinical Chemistry in Lausanne, Switzerland, researcher Paul Kouchakoff found that the body recognizes cooked foods as harmful invaders that need to be eliminated. In simple terms, the white corpuscles (leukocytes) race toward the invasion site (the intestines) as soon as food enters the mouth. This results in an elevated white blood cell count (leukocytosis), which signals an inflamed terrain caused by an attack, in this case in the digestive region.

As it turns out, eating cooked foods never fails to trigger a mobilization of white blood cells. In contrast, white blood cell levels do not increase when raw foods are eaten. Leukocytosis also does not occur when raw foods are ingested with cooked foods.

THE NUTRIENTS TRANSFORMED
BY COOKING

Vitamins

Vitamins are organic substances that the body needs to perform thousands of different operations of building and destroying. All make possible specific reactions at every echelon of the metabolic chains. They are essential to the growth and functioning of all living beings.

Enzymes

All foods consist of vitamins, minerals, proteins, carbohydrates, and lipids, as well as enzymes, which allow the body to better digest and assimilate the food it eats. As it happens, these enzymes become adulterated by cooking. According to nutrition researcher Edward Howell, who has written many books on the subject, the digestive system is then forced to draw on enzymes from the body itself to ensure the digestion of cooked foods.

No organic life would be possible without digestive enzymes. We ourselves have fifteen thousand of them in our bodies, and they serve as catalysts that multiply the biochemical reactions of our digestion. They have the virtue of accelerating chemical reactions without taking part in them while acting at body temperature. Because they are not participants in the reaction, they remain identical at the end of the reaction and ready to react again.

Minerals

Human beings cannot assimilate inorganic minerals because they attach poorly to molecular structures. When processed through a plant, however, they become integrated into a more complex and living molecular construction. In this form, we can assimilate them.

Cooking accelerates the molecular vibration of foods, causing minerals to escape from the complex structures with which they had been combined. These minerals become free and return to their original inorganic state. They can no longer recombine with other substances, like vitamins, enzymes, and amino acids, to build cells. When we consume them but cannot assimilate them, they accumulate, which can cause tissues to harden and arteries to become sclerotic.

Likewise, the minerals found in drinking water are in an inorganic state and cannot be metabolized. They clutter up the kidneys and impede their function.

Proteins

Cooking causes all proteins to coagulate, this is why egg whites become hard and meat shrinks in size during cooking. Coagulation makes them less permeable to digestive juices and leads to gastric hyperacidity. Furthermore, the cooking of meat reduces the bioavailability of its proteins by an order of 60 percent and leaves numerous acidic residues behind. To make up for these amino acid losses, we are advised to eat more protein to ensure that we get the minimum we need to maintain vitality, but this will lead to excess work for the eliminatory organs, which become overburdened by these acidic wastes.

Plant proteins have the advantage of being easily eaten raw and are therefore not altered by cooking. Some good sources of plant proteins include bean sprouts, oilseeds, spinach, certain aromatic herbs, pecans, hazelnuts, and cashews.

Lipids

When heated, the lipids (fats) in oils become adulterated. At temperatures greater than 392°F, fats create new chemical compounds that can be quite toxic. The most visible form is the carbonized rind of meats, which contains cancer-causing substances known as acroleins. When meat and fish are cooked, their fats become oxidized and saturated, requiring a more complicated metabolic process accompanied by overproduction of endogenous cholesterol.

Oilseed crops contain lecithin, an emulsifier of fats, which helps their digestion. When the oils from these crops are grilled, however, the lecithin loses its emulsifying properties.

COOKING METHODS TO AVOID

Cooking at high temperatures (above 230°F and especially 400°F), such as by frying and grilling, clearly increases the production of altered molecules that are indigestible and/or toxic.

Frying

In oils used for frying, the critical factor is the oil's smoke point: the point at which it begins to smoke. This is the temperature at which the lipids in the oil become adulterated and saturated and produce indigestible or toxic (carcinogenic) compounds.

Olive oil reaches its smoke point at 410°F and peanut oil at about 430°F. Oils containing omega-3s are especially fragile at high temperatures. Butter, too, is not a good fat for cooking as its smoke point is low (240°F to 284°F). All other fats (lard, palm oil, coconut oil, and so forth) should be avoided for frying. This will also help you avoid the excessive intake of saturated fatty acids that cause metabolic overload and produce toxins. The connection between these fatty acids and cardiovascular and neurodegenerative diseases has long been common knowledge.

An exception is goose fat and duck fat, which do not possess these disadvantages and can be used to brown potatoes from time to time. These fats are traditionally used in the cuisine of southwestern France. Their high content of monounsaturated and saturated fatty acids makes their lipids quite strong; they have little tendency to oxidize and are resistant to heat.

Grilling

Here, even more substantial precautions need to be taken. When meat has been blackened and carbonized, it has been transformed into toxic products (benzopyrenes and carcinogens). This is especially the case in fatty meats, for which cooking is prolonged and the fat burns beneath the meat being grilled. And those benzopyrenes form whether we are cooking with charcoal or over an open flame. (The same is true for roasted coffee.)

Microwave Cooking

Microwaving, which steals all vitality from food and profoundly alters its molecular structure, causes a directional change of the water molecules more than two billion times a second. It profoundly alters the electron structure of food molecules—with a reduction of electrons—a situation that causes oxidation and cell death. Here is one everyday example: The milk of a baby's bottle that has been heated in a microwave no longer contains proline in a digestible form. The original L-proline has been transformed into D-proline, which is toxic for the nervous system, liver, and kidneys.

BETTER WAYS TO COOK

The cooking methods below preserve the vitality of foods and their nutritional qualities (vitamins, trace elements, and so on).

Steaming over Boiling Water

Advantages

For vegetables that were not grown organically, the steam causes the peripheral cells to release their contents (herbicides, insecticides) into the water of the pot beneath, which will be discarded.

Steaming meat causes its fats to partially melt.

Disadvantages

This method has less respect for vitamins and molecular architecture than steaming food in its own juices; the mineral content is also reduced.

Steaming Food in Its Own Juices

This method can be used for organic vegetables, meats, and fish.

Advantages

It respects the molecular architecture and composition of the minerals and trace elements, and it preserves the majority of vitamins if the foods remain protected from air (no oxidation).

It also maintains the color and flavor of raw foods (the plant cells remain intact).

Cooking in Parchment Paper

This is a reduced model of steaming food in its own juices. The food is placed in its natural state, with seasonings and spices, in greaseproof paper. Avoid aluminum foil, which can allow aluminum particles to get into the food.

This method is essentially used for small fish, seafood, and potatoes.

I would like to remind readers that Leonardo da Vinci, the greatest artist in history, was a vegetarian. This could explain his genius—and the world's best-known painting, da Vinci's *Mona Lisa*.

It would be interesting to write a book that listed all the geniuses who were vegetarians, but for now let's explore the benefits of raw plant foods in relation to Alzheimer's and our olfactory system.

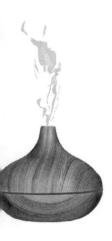

15

Return to the Raw

Establishing an Olfactory-Friendly Diet

THERE IS AN OLD PROVERB that says that, to know where you are going, you must know where you are coming from. If we applied this reasoning to human beings, when observing humanity's evolution and that of our ancestors, the conclusion would have a lot to teach us. Our ancestors were 90 percent vegetarian, with a diet based on fruits and leaves. This explains why fruits and vegetables are so good for our health: we are perfectly adapted to them!

Our earliest ancestors never cooked their vegetables; they followed a raw food diet. History tells us that humans did not master fire until 450,000 years ago. We didn't start cooking food until much later, whether by direct cooking (a rudimentary spit or over hot embers), boiling (in hide containers), or stewing (wrapped in clay). An even bigger question is whether, over that time, our bodies have adapted to cooked foods.

Certainty about anything in this field is hard to come by, and it is difficult to estimate the frequency and intensity of our early ancestors' cooking practices. Given the technical difficulties, it is likely that cooking was far from perfect and reserved for only a small number of foods.

We find some clues from the remote vestiges of the first kitchens.

It seems that the preferred cooking method in our earliest history was not grilling—whether by contact with flame or with embers—but steaming food in its natural juices; the foods were wrapped in large leaves and buried next to a fire or placed in contact with hot stones. This gentle and nontoxic form of cooking was very good at preserving nutrients.

This is why numerous paleontologists and nutritionists have taken an interest in the diet of prehistoric humans (*Homo erectus, Homo sapiens*). The latter were hunter-gatherers from the dawn of humanity until the Neolithic revolution. They ate the meat of the game they hunted, fruits, wild berries, various vegetables (varying in accordance with habitat), and varying quantities of seeds (cereal grains and others). They did not drink the milk of any other animal. They followed this diet for a very long time without any culinary artifice, simply as it was prepared by nature.

Without knowing it, our hunter-gatherer ancestors closely adhered to the values recommended by our modern nutritional experts. Their diet was high in slow carbohydrates (which are favorable for a good energetic metabolism), low in animal lipids, very high in polyunsaturated fatty acids (which are favorable from the perspective of cardiovascular and neurological needs), balanced in cholesterol, very high in dietary fiber (good for proper digestive transit), sufficient in sodium, very high in calcium, and high in vitamin C (antioxidant, anti-scurvy, and favorable for optimum activity).

Today, the enzymes of our digestive tract are still designed for the molecules consumed by our prehistoric ancestors. These enzymes have still not adjusted to the new molecular structures, often quite sizable, that can be found in animal milk, mutated grains, and cooked foods.

INSTINCTOTHERAPY

Our olfactory system is a veritable laboratory. The messages our brain delivers in response to the information brought in by smells are simple and direct: "That smells good." "That smells bad." "I can't smell anything." "I don't like that." In other words, smells tell us "I like" or "I don't like," and in yet other words, "this suits me" (or not) or "this is something my body needs" (or doesn't need).

The simple explanation for this instinct resides in the incredible perfection of our olfactory system, which is connected to a laboratory of sensory analysis that is more powerful than even the most sophisticated modern lab. The information detected by our olfactory bulb is transmitted instantaneously to our brain. The olfactory bulb, stimulated during retronasal smell by mastication and the introduction of saliva, detects and isolates the molecules of a food and transmits information about them to the brain, which analyzes them and logically selects them out of naturally available foods. This approach is in accord with "instinctotherapy."

Our sense of smell, coupled with a laboratory that performs sensory analysis, functions at its best when dealing with raw, pure ingredients like those found in nature and not so well when it is dealing with foods adulterated by cooking. Hence the necessity of giving preference to foods in their natural state.

The range of foods we encounter has evolved considerably since the emergence of an industrial food system characterized by intensive agriculture and transformation of ingredients. But the olfactory system represented by the fabulous software program of sensors and sensory analyzers, initially designed to serve as a compass for *Homo sapiens,* continues to play the same role it has played throughout human history. It has not changed, and this leads to the conclusion that we should distance ourselves from cooking, which places the gustatory system higher than the olfactory system.

THE BASIC FOODS OF A LIVING DIET

At the Heart of Life: Chlorophyll

Chlorophyll is a green pigment that is characteristic of most plants. It is the primary vector of the cycle of life because it plays a role in photosynthesis. All plant life that has any contact with the sun contains some chlorophyll. If there were no chlorophyll, there would be no life on Earth: no plants, no animals, and no human beings.

Its molecular kinship with our hemoglobin has earned chlorophyll the nickname of "plant blood." It is an important supplier of oxygen, an efficient regulator of the acid-alkaline balance, and a blood purifier and detoxifier, all of which are essential for the optimum functioning of our bodies.

Chlorophyll does not survive cooking.

Living foods that are high in chlorophyll include leafy green vegetables, freshwater microalgae (spirulina, chlorella, aphanizomenon), and green juices, particularly wheatgrass juice and that of other grains, whose chlorophyll content has no rival.

Vegetables

Ideally, vegetables in the diet are plentiful, local, and seasonal: black radishes, broccoli, cabbage (red and green), carrots, cauliflower, celery, cucumbers, fennel, kohlrabi, mushrooms, onions, peppers (avoid green peppers, which are not ripe), radishes, red beets, tomatoes (fully ripe and only in season), zucchini, and, of course, all the leafy greens (arugula, chicory, lamb's lettuce, lettuce, spinach, watercress, and the like) and all the aromatic herbs (basil, cilantro, mint, parsley, tarragon, and so on).

Germinated Seeds

Seed germination, which occurs in a moist, warm environment, triggers a powerful burst of enzymatic activity as well as the transformation and multiplication of certain nutrients. Starch is transformed into free simple sugars; gluten, a viscous and insoluble protein that binds starch molecules together, transforms into free amino acids. With vitamins, trace elements, proteins, and enzymes, sprouts are very nutritious and easily digested and assimilated by the body, offering a nutritional and gastronomic contribution of the first order.

A great many seeds can be germinated:

- ✦ Leguminous seeds, like alfalfa (or lucerne), buckwheat, chickpeas, fenugreek, lentils, and mung beans
- ✦ Cereal grains, like barley, corn, oats, quinoa, rye, and wheat
- ✦ Oleaginous seeds, like almonds, flax, hazelnuts, hemp, sesame, and sunflower
- ✦ Vegetable seeds, like arugula, beets, broccoli, cabbage, carrots, celery, fennel, leek, mustard, onion, parsley, radish, spinach, turnip, and watercress

The enzymes developed by germination allow the seeds to self-digest, which breaks down the phytic acid contained in cereal grains and thus makes it possible for the minerals they contain to be digested.

Sprouted seeds allow cellulose intake for people with sensitive intestines to be reduced. Germination enhances the alkalinizing power of seeds and transforms those that are acidic. Soaking and germination are two successive phases of alkalinizing: the germinated seeds boost alkaline levels in the body, they are detoxifying, and they encourage cellular oxygenation.

However, tomato, eggplant, and rhubarb seeds should not be eaten as sprouts; they contain toxic molecules.

Lactofermented Vegetables

Lactofermentation offers us a way to return to raw, live, and natural foods. This ancient food preservation method, spread throughout the world, has regained its former prestige and recognition of its immense virtues with current studies on intestinal flora.

All fermentations—lactic, alcoholic, acetic—result in the transformation of sugars into lactic acid, alcohol, and vinegar, respectively.

Lactofermented foods have been part of the human diet for as far back as we can see. This ancestral and universal practice makes it possible to preserve perishable foods not only without lessoning their vitality but also by galvanizing them. This is a long way from pasteurization, sterilization, and irradiation, all of which devitalize and weaken foods mainly by destroying enzymes and vitamins. The joint intervention of bacteria favorable to health is at work in the process of lactic fermentation. These bacteria can be labeled "probiotic" not only because they strengthen the intestinal flora but also because they enhance the vitality of the food.

I recommend eating lactofermented foods at the start of a meal and in reasonable quantities, for their high content of active principles accelerates their digestion and encourages the digestion of other foods.

Raw sauerkraut and kimchi are the best-known and most common forms of lactofermented foods, but a large number of other foods can be fermented this way, including beets, brassicas (like cabbage and cauliflower), carrots, celery, cucumbers, garlic, green beans, onions, parsnip, peppers, radishes, and turnips. Predigested by the fermentation process, they constitute a supply of nutritious substances that are rich in enzymes, easy to digest, revitalizing, and purifying. Certain fruits, such as papaya, which has powerful antioxidant properties and reinforce our immune system, can also be lactofermented.

Some foods, when fermented, have anti-inflammatory properties and chelate heavy metals. These include:

- ◆ Citrus (lemons and oranges)
- ◆ Edible seaweeds
- ◆ Cereal grains and leguminous plants

Spices, Condiments, and Aromatic Herbs

Spices and aromatic herbs with a particularly high content of active principles, micronutrients, and antioxidants hold a choice position in a live food diet. These include basil, cacao, cardamom, carob, cayenne pepper, chervil, chives, cilantro, cinnamon, cloves, ginger, juniper berry, mint, nutmeg, oregano, parsley, rosemary, saffron, savory, tarragon, thyme, and turmeric, which can be used for seasoning or as a garnish. Of course, preference should logically go to fresh aromatic herbs (enzymes, chlorophyll, vitamins) over dried ones. (And never, under any circumstances, use spices that have been irradiated.)

Garlic is a common culinary ingredient but also has been used for millennia for its antiseptic, antibacterial, and antibiotic properties. Furthermore, it has a beneficial effect on blood lipid balance and is helpful for dealing with cardiovascular problems. Its high antioxidant content makes it a valuable ally in the prevention of aging. It has been shown to be a neural antimutagen, to offer protection for the heart, and to be helpful in reducing cholesterol levels in the bloodstream. When we consume it regularly, we can also benefit from the vitamin B_6, manganese, phosphorus, iron, copper, selenium, and vitamin C it contains.

Fresh Juices:
Vegetable, Fruit, and Wheatgrass

Drinking a single glass of freshly made juice allows us to benefit from the nutrients contained in a large quantity of vegetables. In contrast to many vitamin supplements, fresh juices do not contain any toxic substances. It is important to make sure plenty of saliva is produced when drinking these juices to make the most of all their benefits. Also be sure to choose fruits and vegetables that are organic and fully ripened.

Green juices have major detoxifying properties and should be part of our everyday diet so that we can benefit from their regenerative qualities. Leafy green vegetables, young sprouts, and germinated seeds are very effective at purifying and removing toxins from the bloodstream. In addition to providing an increased quantity of oxygen (because of the chlorophyll they contain), green juices supply minerals, trace elements, proteins, and enzymes. They are very good at restoring health to the body and keeping it in good physiological condition.

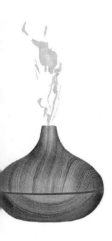

16

Prevention

Tips for Maintaining a Healthy Mental State

TO MAINTAIN a good mental state, you need to supply your brain with

+ Pure water, with few minerals;
+ Carbohydrates, especially slow ones;
+ Vegetable proteins;
+ Nutrients: vitamins, minerals, trace elements;
+ Oxygen;
+ Polyunsaturated fats, preferably EPA and DHA;
+ Antioxidants;
+ Good cerebral circulation with the help of *Ginkgo biloba;* and
+ A Mediterranean diet.

At the same time, pains should be taken to lead a peaceful and harmonious life by

+ Managing stress,
+ Getting good sleep and taking naps when needed,
+ Taking time for yourself and for leisure activities you enjoy,

✦ Keeping your memory fit with intellectual activities, and

✦ Maintaining independence.

MUSIC

Rhythms and melodies possess a calming effect; while music has charms that can calm the savage beast, it is also good for the meninges. In fact, it draws on numerous zones of the brain. It can even permit the construction of new connections between the neurons. As shown by brain imaging techniques, listening to a melody had the ability to animate certain cerebral areas, especially the limbic brain.

Neurobiologists have long known that long-term practice of music can substantially modify neural networks in the brain, including enlargement of the hippocampus. (The work of French professor Hervé Platel has focused on this aspect of brain development.) Because the brain is malleable at any age—that is, it expresses neuroplasticity—it is capable of creating new connections or reactivating those that were less active, giving musicians expanded neuronal resources to draw from. Musicians, in fact, have a greater memory capacity and ability to focus and plan. For these reasons, musical practice could make it possible to delay the appearance of symptoms encountered in neurodegenerative diseases.

In children, music has been shown to enhance their ability to learn to talk and to improve verbal memory, reading, and concentration. According to neurologist and neuropsychiatrist Catherine Thomas-Anterion, "In children who began to learn music before the age of seven, brain plasticity and the impact on other learning seems to go far beyond memory and concerns a good many intellectual aptitudes, namely attention or the organization of speech."

MEDITATION

Whether Buddhism, Hinduism, Taoism, Islam, or Christianity, meditation is present in numerous religious and spiritual practices. Cohabitating at the very heart of Buddhism we find Zen or Zazen meditation (in which attention to proper posture is the high priority), Samatha meditation (for calming the mind), and Vypassana meditation (the practice of clear insight), as described in the earliest spiritual texts. Meditation practice is employed today in therapy through mindfulness (in full awareness) meditations.

Meditation does not consist of "thinking of nothing" or "creating a void" but of welcoming our thoughts and allowing them to pass through without lingering on them and fully focusing attention on the present moment. This makes it possible to regulate emotions and to escape from constant concern about the future (a source of stress) or the past (associated with painful emotions).

Breath is one of the essential components of meditation. Focusing attention on our breath helps us calm our mind and connect more easily with the present moment. In concrete terms, the exercises consist of focusing attention on an object or sensation or, alternatively, the total opposite, focusing instead on everything that surrounds us.

Compassionate meditation aims at focusing specifically on the benevolent love we can hold for others (empathy).

Moreover, for people suffering from depression, meditation has proved to be as effective as antidepressants in the prevention of relapses. Additionally, regular practice will substantially alter cerebral activity, which has a protective effect on the brain. It will develop neuronal plasticity while increasing the density of the tissue of the left prefrontal cortex. This is the part of the brain involved in cognitive and emotional processes as well as the feeling of well-being.

YOGA

Born in India some several thousand years ago, yoga is a discipline for freeing the spirit by mastering movement, rhythm, and breath. It is based on an oral tradition, accompanied by texts like the Yoga Sutras, a treatise in which the sage Patanjali—five hundred years before Jesus Christ—compiled all the then existing knowledge related to this practice. There are several different forms of yoga, with hatha yoga being the most popular form in the West. The United Nations established an International Day of Yoga that is celebrated on June 21.

Hatha yoga is described as a series of postures (asanas), each of which bears a name (Sun Salutation, Cobra, Scorpion, Warrior, and so forth). Performed in an established order, the purpose of these gentle movements (stretches, bends, and twists) is to stimulate the internal organs and provide greater body awareness.

The postures are coordinated with breathing exercises (pranayamas), which allow the development of vital energy and concentration. The session ends with a posture of relaxation or even a period of meditation. The simplest yoga meditation involves repeating mantras silently, to yourself. It is a little like the Hare Krishna devotees who repeat the name of the god Krishna 1,728 times a day.

Yoga practice has a positive influence on stress and anxiety. This improvement corresponds with a significant expansion in one area of the brain, the thalamus, and an increase in GABA neurotransmitters. During the practice of yoga, GABA inhibits the activity of some neurons and stimulates the brain's calming circuitry like a natural anti-anxiety drug. Yoga also reduces levels of cortisol, the stress hormone, which is regulated by the hypothalamus, and increases the production of serotonin, a mood stabilizer.

Practicing yoga two or three times a week thereby has a positive effect on depressive symptoms. Research has shown an improvement in the quality of life, a reduction of stress, better sleep, and a strengthened immune system.

THE PLACE OF PHYSICAL ACTIVITY

Physical exercise is a powerful regulator of brain activity. The more you exercise, the greater protection your brain enjoys. People who exercise often and regularly have a 50 percent lesser risk of developing Alzheimer's disease compared to people who are sedentary.

For this reason, it is a good idea to regularly practice a physical activity of moderate intensity. Try thirty minutes, three times a week; power walking, swimming, jogging, bowling, golf, bike riding, dancing, aerobics, and so forth are all good options.

THE PLACE OF COGNITIVE ACTIVITY

The brain, which is endowed with extreme plasticity, is not a fixed organ. Remember, the cerebral reserve describes, in part, the quantity of available neurons and neural connections, while the cognitive reserve describes the capacity for mobilizing neurons. The goal is to increase the cognitive reserve by a set of stimulations that make it possible to optimize cognitive performance by recruiting other regions of the brain or using new cognitive strategies. The larger the cognitive reserve, the longer we are able to function without any symptoms of neurodegenerative disease appearing.

There are several avenues for activating your brain and enhancing your cognitive reserve:

+ Have projects and goals.
+ Be curious: visit exhibitions, museums, and attend lectures.
+ Do crossword puzzles, jigsaw puzzles, sudoku, and the like.

✦ Play games of strategy: cards, board games, digital games.

✦ Revisit recent events, walks, and encounters in your memory and review the details.

✦ Have conversations and discussions with other people.

✦ Get back into the pleasure of reading and writing: letters, postcards, emails. Keep a diary or write your memoirs.

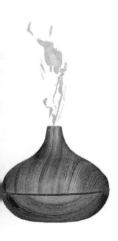

17

We Are
What We Eat

Brain Food Supplements

PHYSICAL ACTIVITY, intellectual stimulation, social interaction, stress management, and good sleep are essential conditions for forming new neurons in the hippocampus and thereby making the fight against Alzheimer's possible. However, these new neurons cannot develop unless we provide our brain with the food it needs. For our memory and cognitive skills to last into an advanced age, the hippocampus needs three basic elements: building materials for the neurons during their developmental phase, energy, and protective agents.

THE ROLE OF NUTRITION

Two aspects can come up when considering nutrition: nutritional deficiencies, which can often be observed among the aged, with negative consequences for the brain, and beneficial nutritional factors that apply specifically to the prevention of Alzheimer's disease.

The risk of nutritional deficiencies increases as we grow older for a variety of reasons. Sometimes it is due to changes in our taste buds and sense of smell that cause us to lose our appetite for certain things. This situation can increase the risk of malnutrition for the elderly and, thus, trigger or worsen a wide range of diseases, including Alzheimer's. These shortcomings can be targeted by the intake of vitamins, enzymes, and fatty acids.

BENEFICIAL FATTY ACIDS

Thinking, moving, communicating, and living naturally are made possible by our cells communicating with each other, exchanging the information that they either produce or receive. The majority of these exchanges are related to the receptor proteins located in the cellular membranes. Each receptor is designed to receive information from a specific messenger (hormones, ions, antibodies, prostaglandins, chemical mediators, and so on).

The encounter between a receptor and a messenger, like the transfer of information into a cell, is shaped by the fluidity of the membrane.

Cellular communication and exchanges are of crucial importance for the body's balance, and for them to happen, the membrane-receptor couple must function perfectly. The membrane is the door to the cell, and the receptors are its keys. The door must be well oiled—which is to say, perfectly fluid. If the fluidity of the membrane leaves something to be desired, exchanges do not occur properly and the cells will suffer consequences.

In terms of nutrition, what allows us to maintain or recover good fluidity of cellular membranes are unmodified polyunsaturated fatty acids in a liquid form, such as those found in fish and plant oils. They are required for neuron development. These fatty acids also regulate our levels of low-density lipoprotein (LDL) cholesterol. We must include them in our diet because the body cannot produce them. They should account for one-third of our daily lipid intake.

Liquid fats from plants are rich in long-chain fatty acids composed of eighteen carbon atoms. They include oleic acid, linoleic acid, and linolenic acid. Linolenic acid is the most unsaturated, with three double bonds. Substantial amounts of it can be found in flaxseed oil, rapeseed (canola) oil, and cold-pressed olive oil.

But there are even longer chains of polyunsaturated fatty acids, composed of twenty or twenty-two carbon atoms, in blue fish like salmon, herring, or eel. They are

+ eicosapentaenoic acid (EPA) and
+ docosahexaenoic acid (DHA).

Both EPA and DHA are omega-3 fatty acids. The modern Western diet is often deficient in omega-3s, leaving us with an imbalanced omega-3: omega-6 ratio, which can pose a health risk (it can cause inflammation). Supplementing with EPA is generally more beneficial for dealing with cardiovascular disorders, while DHA is preferred for protecting cognitive functions. If cognitive disturbances are an issue, take 2 to 3 grams of DHA a day.

Krill oil is quite interesting as the omega-3s it contains are bound to phospholipids (as opposed to triglycerides, as is the case with other fish oils).

Other sources for omega-3s include certain plant-based oils, such as flaxseed oil, olive oil, walnut oil, and rapeseed (canola) oil. They restore cellular membrane fluidity and, in contrast to omega-6s, are anti-inflammatory.

NEUROTRANSMITTERS

The billions of neurons that make up the human brain are connected to each other, and these connections require the presence of chemical substances called neurotransmitters. They exist in large number, and their numbers are reduced by Alzheimer's disease. But there is one that is particularly vulnerable and is weakened in a constant and persistent manner by this disorder. That neurotransmitter is acetylcholine. Cholinergic neurons—that is, those that interact with acetylcholine—ensure the connections between the hippocampus and cerebral cortex, and this neurotransmitter is thereby involved in all the mechanisms of memorization. Researchers estimate that acetylcholine levels inside the brain are already reduced by 40 percent by the time the first signs of Alzheimer's appear.

Anticholinesterase Drugs

Conventional treatments offered to Alzheimer patients are rather disappointing. They essentially consist of medications that increase cholinergic neurotransmission by inhibiting acetylcholinesterase. These anticholinesterase drugs, as they are called, block the action of cholinesterase, the enzyme that breaks down acetylcholine. They are prescribed at the onset of Alzheimer's, and they temporarily improve memory and behavioral problems during the first phases of the disease. However, they have no effect whatsoever on the constant progression of the underlying cerebral deterioration. They can only delay by several months or several years the inevitable course of the disease.

The side effects of the cholinergic medications primarily affect the liver (with an increase of the ALT and AST transaminases), but they also cause nausea, diarrhea, and insomnia, which limits their prescription.

Natural Acetylcholine Supporters

There are newer products that are more effective as well as having fewer unwanted side effects. Moreover, they are natural substances that the body can accept better.

Phosphatidylserine

The phospholipid phosphatidylserine is quite abundant in brain neurons and one of the components of the neuron cell membrane. In Alzheimer's disease, phosphatidylserine levels in the brain are reduced. Several studies have shown that supplementation with phosphatidylserine—which encourages the release of acetylcholine—can improve cognitive function, with improvement in memorization and learning capacity for Alzheimer's patients who have not yet entered a severe stage of the disease.

Effective doses range from 200 to 300 mg a day. Phosphatidylserine can also be found in cruciferous vegetables, soy lecithin, and eggs.

Alpha-glyceryl-phosphoryl-choline

The compound alpha-glyceryl-phosphoryl-choline, also known as alpha-GPC or choline alphoscerate, is an acetylcholine precursor. Once ingested, it transforms into phospholipids and choline, which encourages the synthesis of acetylcholine and phosphatidylcholine. A study has shown that alpha-GPC (1,200 mg daily for six months) significantly improves the cognitive functions of Alzheimer's patients (De Jesus Moreno Moreno 2003).

The most effective dose would be 1,200 mg a day (400 mg three times a day).

Acetyl-L-Carnitine

Acetyl-L-Carnitine is derived from the L-carnitine amino acid. It encourages energy production in the furnaces of our cells: the mitochondria. Acetyl-L-carnitine has other virtues: it purges the mitochondria of the toxic by-products that they have a tendency to collect.

Acetyl-L-carnitine is the cerebro-active version of L-carnitine; it increases the use of glucose in the brain. A meta-analysis of clinical studies confirmed the beneficial effects of supplementation with acetyl-L-carnitine in the treatment of mild cognitive impairment. The participants in these tests took 1,500 to 3,000 mg a day for three to twelve months. Even in centenarians, a reduction of physical and mental fatigue and improvement in cognitive function was observed (Montgomery et al. 2003).

It is recommended to take acetyl-L-carnitine together with alpha-lipoic acid, a mitochondrial fatty acid that plays a role in energy metabolism and has antioxidant properties. Alpha-lipoic acid has been shown to work in synergy with acetyl-L-carnitine.

DMAE

DMAE (dimethylaminoethanol or dimethylethanolamine) is a compound that is transformed to acetylcholine in the body. It acts on the membranes of nerve cells, improving their permeability and resistance to stress.

DMAE has been studied primarily for its possible use in treating the decline of cognitive functions linked to aging. Taking DMAE has been shown to be beneficial in dealing with memory disturbances, lack of concentration and initiative, chronic fatigue, and depression. In the first stages of Alzheimer's disease, DMAE improves motor abilities and vocabulary memory and also reduces anxiety. It has also been used successfully in a variety of disorders and disruptions including attention deficit hyperactivity disorder (ADHD) and memory lapses.

I would like to note here that essential oils (especially rosemary essential oil) also regenerate acetylcholine; see chapter 13.

VITAMINS

Vitamins A (and its precursor beta-carotene), C, and E play a protective role in cognitive health. In people over the age of sixty who are otherwise in good health, memory performance appears to be connected with blood levels of beta-carotene, vitamin C, and vitamin E, and levels of all three are tangibly lower in people with Alzheimer's disease.

B Vitamins

B vitamins are crucial for cognitive health. A deficiency in any of them will lead to mental disruptions, including fatigue, lassitude, vertigo, cramps, tingling, irritability, excitation, and problems sleeping. Generally speaking, the B vitamins can be found in cereal grains, brewer's yeast, whole grain bread, meat, some vegetables, and beans (lentils, peas, chickpeas, fava beans, white beans).

Vitamin B deficiencies are common in the elderly; half of them may have a deficiency in one or more of this vitamin group. As much as 15 to 30 percent are deficient in B_6, 10 to 30 percent in B_9, and 11 percent in B_{12}.

The majority of the B vitamins (except for B_{12}) are at least partially synthesized by the intestinal flora, then stored and metabolized for the most part in the hepatic cells. The restrictive factor that hinders absorption of these vitamins is leaky gut syndrome. This condition, as discussed earlier in this book, is primarily caused by certain medications taken over a long period of time, but some foods (gluten, dairy products) can also be the culprits.

Vitamin B_{12} is the sole B vitamin that is found exclusively in animal products (liver, herring, dairy products). Oddly enough, human beings are the sole animal species that are not able to rely on the endogenous synthesis of this vitamin by the intestinal bacteria.

Vitamin B_3, or niacin, has a strong affinity with the nicotinic acetylcholine receptors by virtue of its proven neurovascular effect. It also mobilizes calcium and offers polyunsaturated acids and LDL protection from oxidation. Among other things, vitamin B_3 is responsible for repairing DNA strands at the same time that it sends calcium (via ADP ribose and inositol) into the intracellular milieu. Finally, it is the sole vitamin directly involved in the mechanisms of phagocytosis, antigens, and the elimination of free radicals.

Vitamin B_6 is a nerve center that allows the synthesis of almost all neurotransmitters; its deficiency is responsible for hyperhomocysteinemia (or better, oxidized hypercysteinemia), which is a prop for all forms of oxidative stress. (In fact, an elevated level of homosysteine indicates a deficiency of vitamins B_3, B_6, and B_{18}, a.k.a. choline.) Moreover, because of its value in metabolizing proteins, vitamin B_6 is involved in the architecture, integrity, and functionality of the genome. It ensures

+ the synthesis of almost all neurotransmitters, including GABA, serotonin, dopamine, noradrenaline, adrenaline, and even acetylcholine; and
+ the catabolism of homocysteine (connected to vitamins B_9, B_{12}, and C).

Vitamins B_9 and B_{12} are combined with the immunomodulatory team of "tryptophan–vitamin B_3–calcium–vitamin B_6." Once Alzheimer's disease is seen to be a xeno- or heteroimmune pathology, this immunomodulatory combination becomes essential.

Vitamin B_9 plays a role in the protection of nerve cells and the manufacture of red blood corpuscles. It permits the renewal and oxygenation of cells as well as the synthesis of neurotransmitters. It can be found in eggs, liver, green vegetables, lentils, spinach, corn, and chestnuts.

Vitamin B_{12} is essential for the proper functioning of neurons, the synthesis of proteins, and the manufacture of red blood corpuscles. It can only be found in animal products: fish, oysters, winkles (snails), liver, and kidneys, among others. A diet that is poor in vitamins B_9 and B_{12} increases the risk of brain atrophy or Alzheimer's disease.

We should remind ourselves that magnesium is essential for transforming all the B vitamins into active coenzymes.

Vitamin E

Vitamin E is the generic name given to a family of compounds that consists of two groups: the tocopherols and the tocotrienols.

Vitamin E is an antioxidant that is soluble in fat (or lipids). As it happens, the brain has very high levels of fat. However, some precautions are called for when taking high doses of vitamin E, as it increases blood fluidity. Opt for a natural vitamin E over a synthetic version.

TRACE ELEMENTS

These are chemical elements that our bodies are not able to produce on their own and that we require only in extremely small quantities for our metabolism. They are iron, iodine, copper, selenium, zinc, and lithium. A deficiency in a trace element can lead to progression of Alzheimer's. At the same time, an excess of certain trace elements can produce the same effect. It is therefore necessary to monitor dosages for supplementation.

Selenium

Selenium plays a role in the metabolism of thyroid hormones. It is an important antioxidant. In the brain, it deactivates chemically aggressive metabolites and also reduces inflammation. Moreover, selenium helps to partially neutralize heavy metals like lead, cadmium, and mercury, whose potential for catabolic damage are well known.

Coconut oil is a good source of selenium, as is sesame oil, though the latter can be allergenic.

The estimated dosage required lies between 100 and 200 mcg (µg/L) daily.

Zinc

The essential trace element zinc is used in all metabolic processes. It blocks excessive release of glutamate and thereby protects the hippocampal neurons from poisoning. A zinc deficiency will inhibit neurogenesis in the hippocampus, which can cause depression and prostate problems and encourage prediabetes.

Our bodies can store only a few grams of this element in our bones, muscles, hair, nails, and skin. Concentrated levels of zinc can be found in squash seeds, oat flakes, wheat bran, lentils, and crustaceans.

The estimated dosage required is 15 to 20 mg daily.

Lithium

The light metal lithium stimulates neurogenesis in the hippocampus and acts as an antidepressant. It neutralizes the excessive release (and therefore collection) of beta-amyloid. Its therapeutic effectiveness against Alzheimer's disease has been demonstrated. Our foods contain very little lithium. Take it in the form of lithium orotate capsules or lithium drops.

Organic Silicon

Silicon has a considerable effect on connective tissue, which strengthens all tissue and organs. It can be found throughout the body, especially in connective tissue, tendons, ligaments, skin, and arteries and veins.

Silicon reinforces the immune defenses. Its anti-inflammatory action accelerates the healing process. Thanks to its multiple actions, it delays aging of the tissue and the brain. It also allows the fixation of water in our cells.

The support tissue inside the brain contains silicon, which makes it possible for the nervous system to stay balanced. Furthermore, silicon chelates aluminum, causing it to precipitate, which offers the brain an additional layer of protection.

The human body cannot metabolize the mineral silica; only organic silica, processed through plants, is capable of being metabolized. It can be found in plant fibers, horsetail (the plant), algae, lithothamnion (an algae), and whole grains.

AMINO ACIDS

Proteins consist of molecules called amino acids. They are indispensable as a source of energy and for replacing dead cells and form part of the composition of all the constituents of the body.

There are twenty different amino acids, of which nine are essential, meaning they are not manufactured by the body and must be provided by diet: histidine, isoleucine, leucine, lysine, methionine, phenylalanine, threonine, tryptophan, and valine. The other amino acids can be synthesized by the body. We find amino acids in the ideal proportions for satisfying the body's requirements in eggs, cow's milk, fish, cheese, meat, soy, brewer's yeast, wheat germ, whole grains, and pollen.

"Complete" proteins contain all of the essential amino acids. Other proteins are labeled "incomplete." Since most complete proteins derive from animal products, a person following a vegetarian or vegan diet will likely need to be sure that it includes brewer's yeast or soy protein. Also, by combining foods with incomplete proteins and foods with complete proteins, we can optimize our amino acid intake.

Examples of ideal combinations:

+ Brewer's yeast and vegetables
+ Rice and green peas (as in Cantonese fried rice)
+ Beans and corn (or corn tortillas)
+ Rice and lentils

Tyrosine

Tyrosine, one of the nonessential amino acids, forms the black pigment melanin when it oxidizes. It is an essential element for chemical reactions that produce the neurotransmitters dopamine and noradrenaline, which are important in mental activity (initiative and seeking pleasure).

Supplementation with tyrosine has been found to help some people who suffer from depression.

The suggested dosage is 500 to 2,000 mg daily.

Tryptophan

L-tryptophan, which is the only biologically active form of this essential amino acid, is often taken for its analgesic, calming, and antidepressant effects. It is a precursor to serotonin, a hormone whose effect is very helpful for soothing mental tensions (depression). Serotonin also plays a role in the synthesis of melatonin, a hormone that has very positive effects for people who have trouble sleeping. L-tryptophan can be found in grains, beans, some nuts, eggs, and soybeans.

It is a good idea to avoid carbohydrates before one o'clock in the afternoon (especially avoid pastries in the morning). They neutralize tryptophan first, then serotonin, melatonin, and leptin, which all depend on tryptophan.

Phenylalanine

The essential amino acid phenylalanine is a precursor for tyrosine, which plays a fundamental role in the management and mental calming of the body (antidepressant). It can be found in oats and wheat germ.

Taurine

Taurine, derivative of cysteine (a sulfur amino acid), is naturally present in the body. The major role of taurine consists of, during an episode of stress, regulating the adrenaline released by adrenal glands and the noradrenaline released by the nervous system. Its activity is close to that of GABA, a modulator of the nervous system, which inhibits the central dopaminergic system and thereby helps with regulating things such as appetite, sleep, and memory.

Methionine

Methionine is one of the essential sulfur amino acids. It has the ability to chelate some heavy metals and possesses properties that reduce cholesterol deposits in the arteries, elevate red blood cell counts, and fight oxidation.

It can be found in eggs, nuts, corn, rice, and grains.

OXYGEN FOR THE BRAIN

Physical exercise is excellent for achieving maximal breathing capacity and oxygenation. Movement makes it possible to dislodge secretions that have become fixed in the bronchia, which helps improve pulmonary ventilation. We have seen that sleep apnea, which can lower blood oxygen levels, is more frequent in Alzheimer's patients, indicating oxygen's fundamental role in providing energy to the brain.

A good supply of ionized air, such as what we would find in forests with pine trees, in the mountains, and by the sea, creates a sense of well-being. There are also devices such as the Bol d'air Jacquier, created by René Jacquier, that offer balanced oxygenation for people living in polluted environments. This device generates volatile peroxidized terpenes extracted from organic turpentine essential oil (extracted from the resin of *Pinus pinaster*). These peroxidized terpenes are inhaled and then integrated with hemoglobin. The unstable group formed of the hemoglobin, pinene, and oxygen releases this oxygen at a cellular level more efficiently than hemoglobin itself.

Because it optimizes our entire metabolism, this method benefits every function of the body.

The effects, which have been observed over the half century since its creation, can be summed up in the following points:

◆ Substantial increase in vitality and recuperative abilities
◆ Development of immune defenses

✦ Optimization of hormonal and nerve functions

✦ Optimization of cardiopulmonary functions

✦ Improvement in lipid and cholesterol levels

✦ Delay of symptoms of aging

✦ Support against diseases of civilization (cancers, Alzheimer's, AIDS, thrombosis, and so on)

✦ Optimization of athletic performance

✦ Detoxification of environmental pollutants

It should be noted that even better results have been found by combining this machine's benefits with supplementation of the trace metals manganese, cobalt, and iron, which are decomposers of peroxides, magnesium chloride, and vitamins A, C, and E.

The device is portable, attractive, and very easy to use. Use it for breathing for two to four minutes twice a day (depending on the device—there are four different models).

Kaqun Water is another option as it contains five times more oxygen than tap water. It is recommended to add some vitamin C (two tablespoons of liposomal vitamin C) to each bottle.

ENZYME THERAPY

An enzyme deficiency can be seen in many senior citizens. As discussed in chapter 14, enzymes are catalysts for almost every single chemical reaction in the body. In most cases they help with digestion or encourage chemical reactions inside the cell. Without their action, proteins, carbohydrates, fats, vitamins, and minerals would be nothing but inert building elements.

Because the food preservation procedures of the modern world destroy a large portion of enzymes, supplementation can be helpful.

Because the intestinal absorption rate of enzymes is 30 percent at best, the quantity must be high to achieve a healing effect. They must be taken with plenty of water and between meals. Supplements containing all the digestive enzymes are recommended in cases of difficult digestion.

As for dosage, follow the manufacturer's instructions, which are generally two capsules two times a day, before meals.

THE ESSENTIAL PLANTS

Turmeric

Turmeric has anti-inflammatory effects and offers protection for nerve cells. But curcumin, its active principle, functions less well when extracted and presented in the form of tablets—only a tiny part makes its way into the brain. Curcumin's problem is its bioavailability: you have to ingest at least 8 grams to see any effect. For this reason, forms that are more bioavailable have been released in the market recently. One of the means of increasing curcumin's bioavailability is to combine it with pepper and fats.

Curcumin's neuroprotective virtues are more visible if we consume turmeric with fish oil. The curcumin and DHA (the active principle of fish oil) could curb the development of Alzheimer's disease.

In 2012, a Chinese research team showed that an intake of curcumin reduced mitochondrial dysfunction resulting from beta-amyloid plaques and protected them from oxidative stress (Huang et al. 2012).

Look for supplements with a standardized extract base that is 95 percent curcurminoids. The dose that seems to be most effective is 200 to 400 mg of standardized extract.

I recommend curry that contains turmeric, two kinds of pepper, and ginger.

Ginkgo

Ginkgo biloba is an extraordinary tree. It is one of the oldest trees in the world and has existed for millions of years. It has survived all the cataclysms known to have occurred throughout history and also is extremely resistant to pollution.

With respect to the brain, its effectiveness no longer requires demonstration. It improves the alertness of elderly people and helps with functional disturbances like vertigo and headaches, but it can be especially important for addressing the symptoms of senile dementia and Alzheimer's disease.

It is especially valuable in prevention. It improves memory when there is a secondary impairment due to age, cerebral vascular insufficiency, and depression. Above all, Ginkgo protects the brain by providing a powerful vascularizing effect and therefore improving the supply of glucose and oxygen it absolutely requires. It acts on the level of microvessels and is a good antioxidant for cardiovascular problems.

Ginkgo is ideally taken as a mother tincture (250 ml vial): forty drops twice a day for two months, stop for one month, then repeat for one month.

Green Tea

Green tea sourced from Asia has high levels of epigallocatechin (EGCG), which is very effective in neutralizing the excess free radicals that can cause us such great health problems. EGCG also inhibits the processes that are specific to Alzheimer's. Even the simple act of drinking green tea regularly reduces levels of toxic beta-amyloid deposited in the hippocampus, the result of which is improved cognitive functioning.

Though we know that green tea has both healing and preventive properties, good sources are important; some batches of matcha tea have been found to be contaminated with aluminum.

Mountain Tea

Mountain tea, prepared from the Balkan plant *Sideritis scardica,* is traditionally used to prevent age-related cognitive problems. Modern studies have confirmed its use as a potent treatment for Alzheimer's symptoms, finding that it removes toxic beta-amyloid (Hofrichter et al. 2016).

Ashitaba

Scientists are often skeptical of folk remedies, but some are very effective. Ashitaba is an example. This member of the carrot family is traditionally attributed with numerous virtues throughout Japan. Research has shown that one of its constituents has an anti-aging effect and promotes autophagy, the physiological mechanism for cleaning and recycling cells (Carmona-Gutierrez et al. 2019). Together, these functions make ashitaba useful for neurodegenerative diseases like Alzheimer's and Parkinson's.

AUTOPHAGY

The word *autophagy* leaped out of the world of science and into the headlines on October 3, 2016, when the Nobel Prize in Physiology or Medicine was awarded to Japanese biologist Yoshinori Ohsumi for his work on this bodily function. It is mainly to Ohsumi's work that we owe the discovery of the genes involved in autophagy.

The term comes from the Greek *auto* (self) and *phagy* (to eat): "eat yourself." Autophagy helps cells cleanse, renew, and defend themselves. It is a fundamental cellular process that allows the body to eliminate and recycle intracellular components as well as trap and destroy invasive microorganisms like viruses and bacteria.

Electroacupuncture for Autophagy

While it may come as a surprise, electroacupuncture (electronic stimulation of acupuncture points, without needles) is capable of stimulating autophagy and improving the health of Alzheimer's patients. At least, that is the conclusion of a study conducted by researchers working with a rat model of Alzheimer's disease (Guo et al. 2016).

The researchers used electroacupuncture to stimulate two points on their rat subjects for a period of several weeks: GV20 (Governing Vessel 20) and BL23 (Bladder 23). GV20, located on the top of the head between the ears, is used in acupuncture mainly to relieve headaches, eye problems, irritability, insomnia, tinnitus, epilepsy, trouble concentrating, and memory lapses. Stimulating GV20 improves all cognitive functions in general. BL23, located on the bladder meridian in the lumbar region of L2 and L3, is used to treat a number of health problems, mainly a lack of energy, loss of libido, lower back pain, ocular problems, and urinary problems, as well as problems with concentration and memory.

The study showed conclusively that the electrostimulation of these points activated greater activity of beclin-1, a protein coding gene connected with autophagy, and the researchers also observed better elimination of beta-amyloids and an improved capacity for learning and remembering in their subjects.

Autophagy plays a major role in

✦ maintaining cellular balance through its catabolic effects (breaking down intracellular elements that have become worn or are present in excess quantity) and anabolic effects (recycling and reshaping elements that have been broken down);

+ energy metabolism, mainly by preserving the viability of mitochondria;
+ immune system surveillance (capturing, sequestering, and destroying germs); and
+ adaptation and survival of cells subject to stress (because of nutritional deficiencies, for example).

We can quickly grasp why a reduction of the autophagy process can have adverse consequences for health. In fact, certain pathologies are closely connected to poor functioning of the autophagy process, including neurodegenerative diseases (Parkinson's, Huntington's, Alzheimer's), cancers, metabolic diseases, infectious diseases, and so on.

In the case of Alzheimer's, we can see the reduction of the autophagy process during the initial stage of the disease in the accumulation of beta-amyloid protein in neurons. This protein is not harmful in itself, but it becomes a threat from the moment its elimination cannot be performed correctly.

It may be possible to stimulate autophagy through diet and nutritional therapy, without resorting to pharmaceutical medications. This could be an interesting path to follow because the many unwanted effects generated by synthetic molecules often makes their use a tricky proposition.

Many nutrients have demonstrated their ability to inhibit the mTOR signaling pathway, which regulates autophagy, thereby having a positive effect on autophagy activation. We can divide them into "green" and "non-green" categories:

+ Green nutrients: curcumin (from turmeric), resveratrol (from red grapes and red wine), EGCG and gallic acid (from green tea), punicalagin (from pomegranates), sulforaphane and diindolylmethane (from cruciferous vegetables)

◆ Non-green nutrients: omega-3s (like EPA and DHA from fatty fish), vitamin D (also from fatty fish)

If it were necessary to pick just one of these nutrients for supplementation in preventive treatment for Alzheimer's, it would unquestionably be vitamin D.

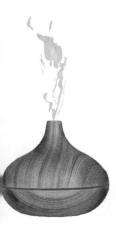

18

Navigating Alzheimer's Disease

A Guide for Families and Caregivers

THE ILLNESS of a family member will overturn the entire structure of a relationship that has been woven together over the years. This disarray is even more profound when the illness is Alzheimer's disease, against which we can fight but never win, and gives birth to a world of misunderstandings and questions.

All families live with their own unique experiences and possibilities. Relations inside the family change, conflicts can burst out of the past or burst up anew, or the family might find itself more tightly knit than ever. Life goes on, but we fear that, sooner or later, it will turn into the Stations of the Cross. The moral suffering felt by the family is made more intense by their long history with the affected family member. Some of the patient's behaviors are manageable, but others have the potential to surprise or destabilize the family milieu.

The moral discomfort can be mitigated by an understanding of how this disease develops. Alzheimer's disease involves the patient and his or her whole family. It turns many situations that seemed settled upside down and brings back to the surface troubling situations that were thought to be resolved. It is impossible to imagine just how oppressive this can be as an everyday reality.

The intellectual, emotional, and relational life of patients doesn't come to a stop at the onset of the disease, and they will react in accordance with the disorder's intensity and their knowledge that their means to fight it are diminishing with time. The greatest value of an early diagnosis is that it allows everyone involved to get used to managing the situation before it has reached a critical point. When the context becomes more difficult, it is necessary to establish a way to handle matters that can head off destabilizing situations. In fact, lack of knowledge about the effect of the disease on our own psyche and that of other caregivers can breed many misunderstandings.

Alzheimer's disease must be understood as an assemblage of cognitive impairments and emotional and relationship disruptions. It will change the way patients think, a change that is more or less profound depending on the stage of the disease. It alters how they relate to the world, to themselves, and to others.

ENTERING THE PATIENT'S WORLD

In its earliest stages, patients are lucid and autonomous. They can go out by themselves, take public transportation in familiar areas, drive a car, and continue to assume the bulk of their daily chores. They speak normally and can express their ideas and feelings. Their social behavior is normal—so normal that people who see them may doubt they are ill.

While life is almost totally normal over the course of these first years, some difficulties appear early and it is necessary to know them to prepare for them appropriately. Other difficulties that begin to gradually appear are going to shake the foundations of everyday life.

Communication permits constant interaction between the person speaking and the person listening: our speech, our attitude, the tone of our voice will modulate, consciously and unconsciously, based on the reactions we see in the person with whom we are talking. With Alzheimer's patients, their feeling of identity will become increasingly dependent on the image we reflect back to them and which is reflected by the other people with whom they have contact. It is therefore imperative to make sure to maintain this representation as much as possible.

Don't be surprised, for example, if their behavior sometimes reminds you of that of a child. It is very necessary to avoid infantilizing or overprotecting our loved ones with Alzheimer's, as this will contribute to the decline of their feeling of who they are and their self-esteem. On the other hand, everything that can reinforce what made them who they are (reminders of events you've shared together, family photos, highlights of their personal qualities) should be made the chief focus of conversation.

Because our loved ones may have difficulty understanding the words or meanings of what we tell them, it is necessary to take some precautions when speaking to them so as to minimize misunderstandings. If they seem to find it hard to understand us, we can verify first that they are hearing us correctly, because hearing impairment is frequent among the aged and complicates their understanding of speech.

Alzheimer's disease is very different and unpredictable from one person and another. Patients may encounter some problems while being spared others. But generally speaking, the attitudes of the people around them have a direct and significant effect on them. Increasing family members' aptitude to interact with patients can extend their capacity to get home care and improve their quality of life. It is essential, on the other hand, to obtain as much information as we can about the problems connected to this disease. This can help us find solutions, better anticipate problems, and bolster our decisions.

As the disease progresses, exchanges with our loved ones will become increasingly laborious and force us to decipher what they wish to tell us. We will also have to learn how to speak to them so they understand us. But why should we continue to communicate with Alzheimer's patients? It would be easy enough, once the diagnosis has been delivered, to simply conclude that these patients are no longer in possession of their faculties and any further communication will be useless. But these exchanges remain essential and healthy. These victims of old age and disease remain our close family members even when illness has altered their intellect. Good communication makes good socialization possible and offers a gratifying compensation for the helper; it also postpones institutionalization. We can help patients make their way through this challenging situation by encouraging all kinds of communication in an atmosphere of warmth and kindness and avoiding situations doomed to fail. We can treat the affected family member like a true conversational partner by speaking to them, listening to them, dialoguing with them, and responding to the messages they have to give.

Understanding

Little by little, we will begin to have to interpret what the patients say to us, for they will have trouble finding words, and the words they use will not always correspond to what they want to tell us. They could use one word instead of another ("pass me the salt" instead of "bread"), mispronounce words ("natlin" for "napkin"), or give them an unusual or even opposite meaning ("no" for "yes"). As incoherent as their words may appear, they have a meaning that we must decipher based on context, expressions, gestures, and regard. It is helpful to verify with our loved ones that we really understood what they meant to say by restating the phrase ourselves.

We must never show any signs of disapproval through words, facial expression (or body language), or attitude. We must never show impatience, even if we feel inside as if we have taken all we can take. We must not put any pressure on them, interrupt them, or jostle them when they are speaking. When they are aphasic or their reason is stuttering, we must show even more receptiveness. When a heavy silence drags on, we can come to their help with expressions that help them pick up the thread: "Yes?" "Then what?" "Are you sure?" If they are struggling to express themselves, we can fill the void before irritation takes them over by improvising on what they are trying to say or by suggesting to them the sentence they are looking for.

We should not forget that our loved ones have just as much trouble understanding our messages as they do formulating their own. In certain situations, when they cannot express their thoughts through words, they will reveal them through behavior. This is why an apparently deviant form of behavior (agitation, aggressiveness) can become the sole possible means for patients in a given situation to respond to messages that seem muddled to them. Often forms of behavior that have been labeled "behavioral disorders" are only manifestations of an intention or a response to a message that was badly interpreted.

So we must get used to speaking with our bodies early, to accompanying our words with gestures that make their meaning more explicit and express kindness, and to touch our loved ones if they do not show reservations about it. This is gestural work in general and more specifically facial expression.

Empathy

According to neurologist Dr. Jean-Pierre Polydor:

> Empathy is the ability to imagine what others are feeling, their feelings and emotions, without feeling them yourself. We draw a distinction between empathy and sympathy, which is the ability to understand the feelings of another, but with a component of sharing them and personalized compassion; sympathy is based on our emotional relationship with the one who is the object. Empathy is neutral knowledge, unrelated to the relationship we have with the

person who is the object (detachment). Empathy involves an intellectual distancing aimed at understanding the emotional states of others, while sympathy is the sharing of feelings. (Polydor 2009)

Validation therapy (therapy using empathy) aims at improving communication with dementia victims at any stage of the impairment's development. In fact, the difficulty patients have with expressing themselves and with comprehension are particularly frustrating and destabilizing for the patients and those around them. The interventions of validation therapy consist of identifying the emotions patients can express and reinforcing them with communication techniques that use both verbal and nonverbal methods (gestures, postures, mimicry).

Emotions

The souvenirs held in our episodic memory are indicated by an emotion. This is why we prioritize the use of photos, aromas, movies, and songs depending upon their ability to evoke an emotionally charged event. The aide who spends time with a patient on a daily basis and knows their personal history well is the person best able to find the inspiration for triggering an emotion.

These evocations are also the pretext to express, recount, sing, move, and mimic the gestures of the patient's job, a favorite sport, and even dancing.

By helping our loved ones rememorize certain old memories, we encourage the emergence of others. We can tell them stories about their life to help them rediscover, through this conquest of identity through their own story, what is called narrative identity. We can speak with certainty here: the senses, the emotions, and stimulation of the sense of smell are the best therapies.

When the End Is Near

"Facing the absolute, all fears are left behind, all passions are soothed, conflicts and recriminations are doomed to disappear before this unfathomable truth—passage into a world about which we would never know anything," Dr. Polydor says.

Attending the last moments of a person at the end of their life is a difficult ordeal to manage. It is difficult for doctors, for health care personnel, and for everyone, but especially for the families.

Death often comes as a terrible physical disaster, which can seem like a shocking agony for overly emotional or sensitive individuals who have not prepared themselves for it. Then again, the end of life can transpire quite peacefully, and family members can see their loved one go out like the tiny flame of a candle and experience this trying time with a blend of sorrow and relief.

The choice is a personal matter, but at no time should a single caregiver, relative, or friend condemn themselves for not having the courage to face the end. We can take into consideration our inability to face certain forms of death from the standpoint of the absolute that we are all poor souls confronting our weaknesses.

OVERALL CARE MANAGEMENT

As we've seen throughout the book, a care protocol for Alzheimer's that is based on the pharmaceutical approach doesn't work; its remedies are not only minimally effective but also have enormous negative side effects. But the objective of the many techniques of health care management that do not follow the pharmaceutical approach is not simply to keep the patients occupied. Theater, music, painting, olfactory therapy—these and other sensorial experiences are key to preserving the cognitive reserve. When establishing such an approach to care, it should be adapted as best it can to the needs of each patient. I recommend that you turn to qualified caregivers who can attempt to rebuild cerebral circuitry, mend ailing brains, calm fears and anxieties, restore pleasure, and recover self-esteem, while at the same time letting patients keep their dignity.

Helping the Helpers

Millions of people worldwide are supporting a dependent relative and often at the expense of their own health. However, there are pathways for getting out of this vicious circle. People who take care of a chronically ill relative often neglect their own needs—this is the weakness of a caregiver. If you are a caregiver, it is important to give yourself some time to yourself. You may also be able to find institutional support systems that you can turn to for getting a break. France, for example, has laws in place that give those who care for the elderly not only the right to a break but also access to professional health care organizations for assistance.

Support for Helpers
after the Patient's Death

The helpers are themselves going to greatly need help after the death of the person they have been assisting. They will need support and community. They will feel relief, both for the patient, who has come to the end of their suffering, and for themselves, who are exhausted and empty. And they will feel guilty for feeling that relief. As Dr. Polydor notes:

> They are also experiencing an empty feeling, a great emptiness after years of constant, even excessive demands that took up all their time: what to do now? Life had been given a meaning by their devoted service; they had found a grail, a devotion to a cause by taking care of the patient, or going to visit them, thinking of them, and managing the thousand little problems. And now what was foreseen for so long has finally happened and nothing can be as it was before.

Once the shock of the death has passed, a kind of emotional disorientation takes hold. Close relatives go through a period of emotional anesthesia during which they feel annihilated.

This second stage does not last long. They will quickly realize, usually within several weeks, when they have returned to their normal life, that they had become accustomed to shaping their lives based on that of the patient. They were completely invested in their caregiving role. What new feelings do they now have? What new meaning can they give their lives?

The friends and family members of caregivers grieving the loss of their patient can help them be resilient by telling stories of the happy times of the patient's life, the funny moments, or the valorizing episodes of their life together as a couple (if the caregiver was the patient's spouse, as is often the case)—all told without bitterness but with plenty of laughs and smiles. In this way, the illness that dominated the end of the loved one's life will be set inside a more harmonious unfolding in which everything was not sad.

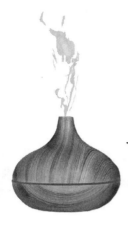

Writing a New Page
of Medical History

ALZHEIMER'S DISEASE is mentioned in the media with increasing frequency, but it is still not considered just another disease. Despite the harshness of the diagnosis, one of the challenges we have to meet is to change the way this disease is perceived and stigmatized for all its negative aspects.

Thirty years ago, Alzheimer's disease was not yet worrisome. Today, it is ravaging the aging populations of our modern society, but what is the most alarming is that it is beginning to afflict younger and younger people.

The history of medicine is only an unremitting high-speed chase between the advent of more or less serious illnesses and the solutions that the medical profession puts together to deal with them. This research must be tireless.

There are some who claim that if we subtracted the notion of illness from cognitive decline, the clinical phenomenon would not be of interest to anyone. To the contrary, it should stimulate the abandonment of an exclusively biomedical model and enlarge it with everything that the social sciences and humanities (anthropology and paleoanthropology) can contribute.

Those who assume that the fact of speaking of cognitive aging will cause people to lose interest in the subject seem to forget the symbolic position that the struggle against aging begins to take up in many people's minds. How is it conceivable that a society that invests so much in the cosmetology of preventing the aging of skin would not do the same for aging of the brain? By explaining what is actually going on here and abandoning the fantasy of finding a pill to cure Alzheimer's we can find our way forward.

"Before inventing the treatment, the gods invented the diagnosis!" Here is a saying that the father of modern medicine, Hippocrates, 2,500 years ago, most certainly would not have renounced. Today, this aphorism is more true than ever. This is because the possibilities of making a patient's illness worse by a misdiagnosis are put into evidence every day. The duty to not hurt the patient through the medical treatment given is an important part of the Hippocratic oath, and doctors always feel bound to respect it.

To pose a reliable diagnosis of Alzheimer's today, we have a range of medical imaging procedures (like PET scans), as well as neuropsychological tests. The last parameter, and not the least, is a detailed medical history. This consists of the observation of the patient's antecedents, which is also the basis of diagnosis, and especially to notice a providential sign—namely, problems with the sense of smell. All that needs to be done for that diagnosis is the performance of an olfactory test.

With these techniques at our avail, today it is possible to reach a diagnosis of Alzheimer's at very early stages of the disease—which is to say, even before the patient shows any signs of impairment of their cognitive abilities.

There is also the fact that over the millennia, the enzymatic inhibition created by the advent of a cooked food diet caused the degeneration and gradual involution of the olfactory system, which in turn caused an inhibition of the physiological functions of the sense of smell. This is why the emergence of Alzheimer's disease is the price we pay for compelling our bodies to adjust to an environment that has been profoundly transformed and for which the olfactory and limbic systems are not genetically programmed.

Here's something worth noting: In my approach to treating Alzheimer's, all chemical remedies are relegated to the sidelines. The essential therapeutic strategy can be summed up as emphasizing raw food and essential oils.

Our hunter-gatherer ancestors were robust and thin. They did not experience chronic illnesses like diabetes, cardiovascular diseases, cancers, Alzheimer's, and autoimmune diseases. And contrary to popular opinion, they did not all die at the age of twenty!

"In these cultures, living past seventy was normal, and it was no rare thing to run across octogenarians," says Dr. Michael Nehls in *Guérir Alzheimer* [Healing Alzheimer's].

In the past, arguments have been made that humans could not develop genetic protection against Alzheimer's because the average life expectancy of our ancestors was only about thirty years. These arguments have been shown to be groundless.

Our longevity is not connected to a highly technological lifestyle; it is the consequence of a process of natural selection that goes back to the dawn of time and guarantees us good intellectual fitness into an advanced age. In other words, this process protects us from the deterioration of our intellectual capacities. Right away we have here an essential piece of information for solving the Alzheimer's puzzle: our genome cannot be held responsible for this disease. And if that is the case, wouldn't it be more logical to search for its causes in our modern lifestyle, as it is the sole parameter that has changed in so short a time? The sole factor for which we can blame our genome is that because of its historic programming, it is not equipped to compensate for and manage the consequences of modern life. As Dr. Nehls says:

Numerous studies today have recently corroborated this hypothesis. They indicate that when we alter one or another of the elements of our traditional lifestyle, some of the processes that are then initiated in our brain increase the risk of Alzheimer's. It is not genetic destiny as much as it is cultural changes that are the engine of this disease. And therefore it is no coincidence that Alzheimer's starts in precisely that part of the brain that allows us to acquire our cultural skills.

What was the secret of our hunter-gatherer ancestors? A healthy lifestyle, which was the lot of humanity for more than two million years. Even today, the paleo lifestyle is the only lifestyle for which we are adapted. The remedy is not everything; nature is the best remedy. "Vis medicatrix naturae," said Samuel Hahnemann, echoing the philosopher Hippocrates twenty-three centuries earlier (400 BCE): "Let your food be your medicine."

Medicine could write new pages of its history, pages of authenticity, acknowledging that the functioning of all living beings is clearly holistic and comprehensive.

For several years, professors of medicine have been studying the sense of smell and neurodegenerative disorders in neurology departments and neuroscience labs. Dissertations are now being written on this theme. Essential oil applications are being used in hospitals, nursing homes, and memory care units around the world. Spectacular results have been recorded in thousands of Alzheimer's cases.

What more needs to be said?

IN SEARCH OF CELLULAR TERRAIN PHYSICIANS

All too often, the doctors and neurologists in charge of treatment refuse to let their patients follow a plan based on the causes of the disease despite the proofs that support its implementation. Here again, the system and the doctrine it spreads are at work, not to mention the pressure applied by pharmaceutical lobbies at risk of losing business.

Currently, thousands of patients are being treated successfully by natural treatments like those described in this book, so all competent and courageous therapists should be sufficiently receptive, in their patients' best interest, to at least take a look at this innovative and effective approach.

This form of treatment against Alzheimer's should not be separated from conventional medicine. We can describe this as a holistic or complementary approach, but that amounts to marginalizing the treatment—and from a scientific point of view, this approach should not be considered marginal. Doctors educated in conventional schools should not unthinkingly push aside a therapeutic concept that eliminates, in a targeted and systematic fashion, the causes of a disease. It is true nevertheless that all too often medical interventions can still be unfortunately summed up as a medical treatment of the symptoms as desired by the system upon which our contemporary societies and allopathic medicine are founded. For the medical establishment and for the purpose of taking stock, it is therefore essential to break with established thought and develop a systematic understanding of the facts: the causes of civilization's diseases are generally to be found in our lifestyle, and only by changing our habits can we find true healing.

It is my firm conviction that the sole hope for healing is to be found in the basis of the knowledge presented here and the exceptional results obtained through it.

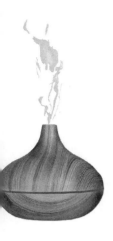

Diseases Akin to Alzheimer's

WHILE ALZHEIMER'S DISEASE is by far the most frequent of the neurodegenerative disorders (it is the cause of seven or eight dementias out of every ten), other disturbances also reveal their presence through cognitive disorders that cause dementia and behavioral changes.

In addition to Alzheimer's, with its increasingly precise diagnostic criteria, neurologists have identified at least two other neurodegenerative diseases: Pick's disease (with it, frontotemporal degenerations), on the one hand, and Lewy body dementia on the other.

Other pathological conditions similar to these exist but are more rare. These related diseases resemble Alzheimer's disease in that they also involve a slow deterioration of brain cells that remains irreversible. These include cerebrovascular disease (second in this group of diseases in terms of frequency after Alzheimer's), frontotemporal disorders, Creutzfeldt-Jakob disease, and Parkinson's disease.

FRONTOTEMPORAL DISORDERS

Frontotemporal degenerations (FTD) represent the second most common cause of degenerative dementia among patients under sixty-five, after Alzheimer's disease.

The signs often appear in younger individuals (under the age of sixty). They can complicate a diagnosis in the sense that the comportment and/or mood of the person has changed while their memory capacity is still excellent. For this reason, the disease can be confused for a psychiatric disorder. In contrast to Alzheimer's, behavioral disorders and not memory problems are dominant.

There are two different kinds of these frontotemporal degenerations: Pick's disease and unspecified frontotemporal degeneration.

Frontotemporal degenerations (often called frontotemporal dementias) are cognitive and behavioral diseases akin to Alzheimer's, although they are much rarer. The incidence in the United States is estimated at a rate of 2.7–4.1 per 100,000.

Contrary to Alzheimer's disease, which affects almost the entire brain, frontotemporal degenerations primarily affect the frontal and temporal lobes, zones associated with personality, behavior, emotions, language, elocution, abstract thought, and motor skills. In the majority of frontotemporal degeneration cases, the cells in these parts of the brain atrophy or die.

In some cases, these same cells become overdeveloped and contain round, argyrophilic "Pick bodies." This finding leads to a diagnosis of Pick's disease, which is a behavioral variant of frontotemporal degeneration. It is the most frequent form of this disorder and shows massive bilateral cortical atrophy.

The condition of the lesions inside the frontal and temporal lobes varies from one individual to the next, which explains why patients will exhibit different signs, sometimes signs that are totally opposite.

Symptoms

Frontotemporal degeneration most often begins between the ages of fifty and sixty-five. It is expressed by behavioral and speech disorders. Social conduct and control of emotions becomes altered.

Behavioral changes can include solitary withdrawal or the loss of inhibitions—that is, individuals lose the ability to control what they say or do. Patients can exhibit a lack of initiative, neglect their personal hygiene, be easily distracted, or continually repeat the same gestures. They can also start eating too much or have a compulsion to put objects in their mouth. Incontinence is sometimes an early sign of this disease. People afflicted with frontotemporal degeneration can become indifferent to the people in their immediate surroundings, display harsh and frequent changes in behavior, or give vent to excessive emotional outbursts. They must often be urged to complete tasks—to get dressed, wash, and so forth. These symptoms sometimes give people the mistaken impression that the patients are suffering from depression.

More rarely, the disease is expressed in relaxed behavior. The patients then appear to be excessively jovial and treat those around them with inappropriate familiarity and a lack of modesty. They also may stop taking care of their personal hygiene.

Frequently, eating habits become problematic. Patients will start eating greedily, shoveling their food down with no manners and often sloppily. These changes may be connected with weight gain at the onset of the disease. It is common for patients' tastes in food to change.

A variety of speech disorders can also affect patients, from difficulty in finding the right word to limited verbal expression and even complete aphasia (muteness). Systematically repeating what other people say and stammering are frequent symptoms. Patients may have difficulty in following a chain of ideas or in holding up their end of a conversation. Their ability to read and write is also affected.

People stricken by frontotemporal degeneration can exhibit a reduced range of facial expression, slowness in their movements, and postural rigidity and instability. Shaking, difficulty walking, frequent falls, and poor coordination can also be common manifestations of this disorder. Patients also lose motor skills and can have problems swallowing.

Memory remains relatively intact, mainly at the onset of the disease, the reverse of Alzheimer's disease. There can be little, if any, problem with spatial orientation. On the other hand, orientation in time can be disrupted.

Tests

There is no single test to identify frontotemporal degenerations. To establish a diagnosis, doctors must detect the characteristic signs of this disease and eliminate all other possible causes.

Neuropsychological tests evaluate the ability to reason, judgment, attention span, memory lapses, and executive and visual-spatial functions.

MRIs or brain scans will reveal atrophy of the frontal and temporal lobes. Brain scintigraphy and PET scans allow more detailed study of cerebral functioning and reveal any anomalies in the frontal and temporal regions.

Laboratory tests and an EEG make it possible to exclude other pathological factors.

A genetic analysis can be suggested if justified by family history. Three genes are most frequently involved.

Treatment

At the current time, there is no known treatment or any effective method for slowing down the development of frontotemporal degeneration. The cholinesterase inhibitors prescribed for Alzheimer's disease are not effective in the treatment of this disease because it affects other parts of the brain. For the moment, the available treatments are concentrated on managing the symptoms of the disease.

PICK'S DISEASE

Arnold Pick first described the characteristics of the disease that bears his name at the end of the nineteenth century. But people continued to confuse it with Alzheimer's until the 1980s, even though articles describing cases of Pick's were regularly published in the medical literature. However, it must be admitted that differentiating a diagnosis between the two is sometimes difficult, especially when we are dealing with an atypical form of Alzheimer's.

Pick's disease begins with behavioral problems that are destined to become the dominant symptoms. These problems can take the form of a protracted apathy, similar to depression, or its total opposite, complete loss of inhibition and any regard for social conventions, abnormal food or alcohol binges, alteration of habits and beliefs, or even a ritualization of behavior (patients become rigid; they don't want to change their behavior and become self-centered).

Memory lapses are frequent, but they remain secondary to the behavioral disorders. Patients have difficulty planning and performing complex activities that require concentration because they are now easily distracted. Problems with language can appear next. Patients are customarily barely aware of these disorders and find it difficult to accept help.

International diagnostic criteria are now available, which allow earlier diagnosis and care management to be implemented.

LEWY BODY DEMENTIA

This disease is similar to Alzheimer's in terms of the age when it customarily shows symptoms (on average, seventy-five) and its frequency (it is estimated to make up from 15 to 25 percent of all neurodegenerative diseases); it is the second highest cause of dementia after the age of sixty-five. Diagnosing Lewy body dementia (LBD) is difficult because, like

Alzheimer's, it can only be done with complete certainty by examining the brain.

Lewy Body Dementia and Parkinson's Disease

Parkinson's disease dementia and Lewy body dementia are similar because they have the same histopathological lesion necessary, but not specific, for making a diagnosis: the Lewy bodies. Though these two degenerative disorders have been described as distinct entities, today they tend to be considered as part of the same pathology, with a motor pole represented by Parkinson's and a dementia pole by Lewy body dementia. In fact, the initial description of Parkinson's referred to motor symptoms outside of any mental impairment. The Lewy bodies were first identified in Parkinson's disease at the beginning of the twentieth century.

Diagnosis

The diagnostic criteria for Lewy body dementia are centered on cognitive changes but have complementary criteria, with three major and eight minor criteria in total.

The major criteria are fluctuations in cognitive function, hallucinations, and the Parkinson syndrome.

The eight minor criteria are frequent falls, fainting, brief losses of consciousness, hypersensitivity to neuroleptics, delirium, hallucinations (auditory, sensory, and olfactory), and, more recently, behavioral issues during REM sleep and depression. A diagnosis of Lewy body dementia requires the combination of one major criteria with at least two minor criteria.

Hallucinations

Hallucinations, which are most often visual, are an essential element in the portrait of Lewy body dementia. They are present in 40 to

75 percent of cases. They can occur several times a week without any triggering factor or specific time. They are most often colorful images of animals and children. These hallucinations can remain with the patient for some time after they initially occur. They are more rarely auditory, and it is only as an exception that they are olfactory, in contrast to Alzheimer's disease, in which 95 percent of such episodes involve the sense of smell.

Trouble Sleeping

Insomnia of all kinds is regularly seen in this disease. Accompanying signs underlie this insomnia: pain (painful cramps and involuntary muscle contractions in particular), restless leg syndrome, muscle spasms, confusion upon awakening, and, more rarely sleep apnea, the consequence of dopaminergic drug treatments. Diurnal hypersomnia can also be seen occurring in this disorder, encouraged by the periods of hyperalertness characteristic of this disease, by the poor quality of sleep at night, and by overprescription of sedatives. At the end of the disease's development, the patient's sleep and waking cycle can be completely disorganized.

The Biological Aspects

Few biological markers have been assessed in diseases with Lewy bodies. Study of the markers of the characteristic lesions—namely, the Lewy bodies—is one of the potential axes. The amount of alpha-synuclein, the constituent protein for Lewy bodies, in the cerebrospinal fluid has been evaluated by some teams studying Parkinson's disease and could be applied as well to Lewy body dementia.

The search for other markers not specific to Lewy body dementia could also be valuable. The amount of hyperphosphorylated tau protein and beta-amyloid protein, for example, in the cerebrospinal fluid could make it possible to determine the links between Lewy body dementia and the Alzheimer's process. Determining these amounts is part of current practice during the first assessment of a possible dementia syndrome.

One interesting element, and a distinguishing feature between Lewy body dementia and Alzheimer's, is that the hippocampus and inner temporal lobe remain the same size in the first disease, whereas reduction in size is an early marker of Alzheimer's disease.

Treatment

The primary treatments are the same whether the disorder is Lewy body disease or Parkinson's disease. The correction of cholinergic and/or dopaminergic deficits is the base of the first treatments made available to victims of Lewy body dementia. An intervention on the glutaminergic system is quite conceivable.

The symptomatic treatment of Lewy body dementia or Parkinson's disease is particularly delicate. In fact, the agents used to treat motor symptoms can have side effects that cause cognitive and behavioral disorders. Furthermore, they have no effect on cognitive impairment. Similarly, the antipsychotics (neuroleptics) that are sometimes necessary for treating psychological and behavioral disorders can also have serious side effects adversely affecting cognitive and motor skills.

Taking antipsychotics (neuroleptics) has the potential to considerably worsen the state of the disease. In fact, many patients lack the enzymes necessary to break down these medications. Any abrupt aggravation of the patient's condition after taking neuroleptics should be addressed by consultation with a specialist.

Better knowledge of the mechanisms involved in the LBD process would make it possible to define a certain number of therapeutic targets. But whatever treatment approach is taken, any therapy can be adapted to include raw foods and essential oils.

SECONDARY
NEURODEGENERATIVE DISORDERS

From 10 to 20 percent of dementia disorders are caused by cerebro-vascular diseases, and for this reason they are called vascular dementias. They are most often due to repeated small strokes called lacunar infarcts. These strokes are caused by the obstruction of small brain arteries due to chronic high blood pressure, atherosclerosis, or old age. They are associated with a lack of irrigation to the white matter of the cerebral hemispheres. These lesions can be spotted easily with a brain scan or MRI, but they are fairly common in the elderly.

Another 10 to 20 percent are mixed dementias. This term designates the combination in one individual of Alzheimer's disease with vascular cerebral lesions. They appear with all the features of Alzheimer's, particularly the problems with recording new memories. The existence of vascular lesions increases the likelihood of dementia and explains the appearance of reflex and motor disorders that are not seen in Alzheimer's disease by itself.

Quite often, the dividing line between the different classifications of dementia can appear vague. Vascular impairment, for example, can be associated with Lewy body dementia. In more than 30 percent of cases, in fact, autopsy of patients with Lewy body dementia reveals vascular lesions. This is why the existence of a cerebral vascular pathology, made visible through morphological brain imaging, does not rule out a diagnosis of Lewy body dementia. It essentially has therapeutic consequence: the two targets, vascular and degenerative, must both be taken into account.

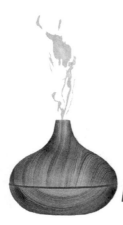

The Nose Knows

Learning from Man's Best Friend

THE SENSE OF SMELL, or olfaction, forms part of our five senses, the others being touch, hearing, taste, and sight. Like taste, smell is a chemical sense that captures sensory information transmitted by suspended molecules. Although the sense of smell is a very primitive function, the mechanisms of the coding of aromas has begun to surrender its secrets.

The detection (and discrimination) of odors is an essential function for survival (identification of food sources, the presence of predators) and reproduction (identification of a sex partner and his or her reproductive availability). This is how we understand the role of this very complex system, which has been preserved over the course of phylogenesis (evolution through time), mainly in humans and mammals.

AN OPTIMIZED MUZZLE

A dog's muzzle corresponds to the human nose. But a dog's sensitivity to odors is from 1,000 to 100,000 times better than that of a human being. This is due primarily to the fact that a dog has fifty million to two hundred million neuroreceptors carpeting its nostrils, compared to the six million in a human's nose.

In addition, when we breathe in air, what we are feeling and what we are breathing in form part of the same flow. Dogs have a membrane inside their muzzles that allows them to separate the airflow into two parts: one part flows toward the lungs, which permits respiration, and the other flows upward, toward the receptor-covered olfactory epithelium, which permits smell. While humans breathe in and out through the same channel, dogs exhale through slits at the sides of their muzzles, which creates whirlwinds of air that strengthen the attraction of new odors into the nostrils.

Dogs also have another active olfactory organ: the vomeronasal organ, or Jacobson's organ, which is present in all mammals but is found in a reduced form in humans. Located behind the incisors above the soft palate, this organ captures pheromones and is therefore useful in the choice of a sexual partner, for example. This olfactory organ would permit dogs to smell the pheromones we emit with particular emotions (sadness, joy, stress, anger) and even to detect diseases or a pregnancy.

The regions of the brain that are dedicated to olfaction are more developed in dogs (and in cats) than in the human being, and they are more apt at identifying odors due to their much more elaborate olfactory system. Their sense of smell is the first alert in the presence of danger, prey, or potential sexual partner.

A dog's nose serves it like a compass intended to ensure the essential—namely, the struggle for survival, reproduction, and adaptation. It was the same for our ancestors during the time before the discovery of fire and cooking.

ANATOMY OF A DOG'S NOSE

A dog's two nostrils are the first exterior elements of its olfactory system. The nasal cavities are particularly well developed: they contain nasal concha and an ethmoidal labyrinth, covered in an olfactory mucous membrane. This olfactory mucous membrane is itself covered by a layer of cells that make up the olfactory epithelium and includes a particularly well-developed nervous system connected to the brain's olfactory bulb.

One advantage dogs, and especially dogs with long noses, have over many other animals is that there is a lot of space in the nasal cavity for a large surface of olfactory epithelium. A German shepherd or Belgian sheepdog, for example, has up to two hundred square centimeters of olfactory mucous membrane, which allows it to house one hundred times more olfactory neurons than a human being.

Note that dogs (along with mice, rats, cows, and opossums) are among those mammals that have approximately one thousand smell receptor genes in their genome. It's 872, to be exact. With this kind of equipment, it's no wonder it performs so highly.

HOW DOES THE DOG'S SENSE OF SMELL FUNCTION?

A dog's unique sense of smell influences the daily behavior of the animal and plays an important role in the hunt for food, when a threat is present, or when it is looking to reproduce. Dogs have two means of perceiving odors: the nasal tract and the retronasal pathway.

The nasal tract has priority. The air breathed by the dog, which carries odor molecules, travels through the nasal cavity. Only 7 percent of the air the dog breathes in reaches the olfactory apparatus.

The retro-nasal pathway is next. Some odor molecules are transmitted directly to the olfactory apparatus during exhalation or in the presence of food or urine. When a dog perceives an odor, it sniffs the source of the odor with several accelerated inhalations and exhalations, which allows the dog to make sure there is better contact between the odor molecules and the olfactory mucous membrane. The retained odor molecules are integrated by the cells of the olfactory epithelium, from where they reach the neurons that interpret the smell and transmit its message to the dog's brain. The animal is then able to interpret its surroundings or even follow a trail. Whether the trail is recent, at a distance, or several days old, this canine function works better than GPS.

THE MECHANISM IN HUMAN BEINGS

Human neuroreceptors, whose life span is four days, are capable of dissolving the odor molecules suspended in the air that has been inhaled and analyzing them. The message is then transmitted to the most archaic part of the brain, which we have in common with all animals. From there, the information is relayed to other cerebral layers to be integrated in the entire perception of a situation. It is then judged as more or less pleasant and compared to past emotional and behavioral reactions before leading to an instinctive reaction or decision.

As we have seen, scent touches the deepest part of our subconscious mind while also mobilizing all brain functions. We know full well that there is nothing like an unpleasant odor to provoke an instinctive reaction of disgust or rejection. Moreover, the olfactory information sent to the two hemispheres constructs a suspension bridge between the logical, rational, and analytic thought of the left brain and the analogical, symbolic, and intuitive thought of the right brain.

THE IMMENSE OLFACTORY
CAPACITIES OF DOGS

A dog's powerful sense of smell is invaluable to human beings, who have used it to their advantage in a variety of ways. It allows dogs

+ to immerse themselves in their environment;
+ to identify the presence of other dogs and other animals, including human beings;

- to pursue reproduction (when a male dog smells the odor released by a female dog in heat);
- to find food;
- to mark their territory, which is also an important means of communication;
- to rescue people when there are earthquakes, avalanches, and other disasters in which they are buried alive;
- to hunt for explosives or drugs; and
- to track down a missing person.

MEDICAL FEATS

People in the medical community should focus their attention on dogs' ability to diagnose disease. Every day, more discoveries are made concerning their ability to identify illnesses like cancer as well as to prevent an imminent attack of epilepsy or hypoglycemia. Some dogs have the ability to identify such attacks fifteen minutes before they happen, which allows their owners to take precautions and prevent any aggravating circumstances surrounding these episodes. In the case of cancer (mainly ovarian, lung, and melanomas), dogs can provide a diagnosis more efficiently and earlier than medical professionals.

Moreover, the presence of dogs (and cats) in nursing homes and memory care centers has a soothing effect on the agitation of patients with Alzheimer's and related disorders. These individuals, who no longer grasp the meaning of words, are being reached through their archaic corporeal sensitivity. The immediate, authentic, and warm contact with an animal gives them profound reassurance. Their heart rates stabilize, and they temporarily enjoy a moment of true connection, accompanied sometimes by fragments of memories that were thought lost once and for all because of the neurodegenerative disorder. The dog they pet can encourage processes of mental attachment that have been totally muddled. For those who are less dependent, the animal can restore a social bond, offering them a break from the terrifying solitude that comes with the seclusion of old age. The animal's life-giving warmth pushes the anguish of death back into the distance.

WHAT IS THE CAT'S STORY?

The sense of smell is particularly useful to cats for several reasons. It is how they identify their territory, that of others (social role), and potential enemies or prey, and, most importantly, smell has an effect on their appetite. With its sense of smell, a cat can quickly distinguish food that is rotting from that which is edible; partial or total loss of the sense of smell can lead a cat straight into anorexia.

These traits show that a cat's sense of smell is clearly more developed than ours. It is, in fact, one hundred times better and is even up to the task of recognizing several thousand odors thanks to its two hundred million olfactory terminals.

When a cat's nose is moist, it means that in the space of an instance it has detected an interesting smell. The moisture comes from activation of the Bowman's glands, which allow a cat to enter into a state of full olfactory evaluation of its environment.

In the same vein, a cat's sense of taste is slightly less developed compared to that of a human being. An adult cat has only 250 taste buds, while an adult human has about 10,000.

THE DOG-CAT-HUMAN ANALOGY

Dogs can sense when a human is scared, but it is not as simple as that. Dogs interpret the feeling of fear thanks to the odors we release. When we are scared, we sweat more and our body language changes; our movements are different and more nervous, and our muscles contract more. A dog can smell this, see this, perceive this, and understand this.

So here is something for humans to ponder and to help them see their cat with new eyes—but therefore differently. In any event, as Arthur Schopenhauer observed, "If you stroke a cat, it will purr; and, as inevitably, if you praise a man, a sweet expression of delight will appear on his face."

When Paul Broca, the French physician who is famous for his categorization of the brain into distinct areas in 1879, identified the olfactory bulb in humans, he noted that its size, in relative volume, was smaller than that of other mammals like the dog or rat. So, he theorized, humans have only an impoverished sense of smell at their disposal. This statement was advanced again by Sigmund Freud, who saw this deficiency of our species as comparable to a mental disease!

Even so, our memory works primarily through our olfactory system. All the events connected to a fragrance are recorded from the first day of our life. Scents can recall images, situations, or experiences we've had and take us back even into our youngest childhood. The sense of smell has no sense of time. Through a fragrance, we can feel a past event again as intensely as we experienced it the first time. This effect, also known as the Proust phenomenon, was described quite well by that author in his *Remembrance of Things Past*. In it, he explains how a childhood memory was brought back to the surface by the smell of a madeleine dipped in tea. At that very moment, this memory gave him a feeling of protection and intense happiness. This scent was transformed into a positive mooring for him.

WHY HAS SCIENCE OVERLOOKED THE SENSE OF SMELL FOR SO LONG?

Smell is a passive sense (you cannot choose what you are smelling), for which reason it was once considered minor and a little bit coarse—furthermore, it is dogs that sniff! In 2014, a study published in the magazine *Science* showed for the first time that a human being can detect a trillion odors (Bushdid et al. 2014). That is immense.

The human genome contains four hundred genes devoted to the sense of smell. As a comparison, there are only four genes for color. It is a very complex palette that has been shaped by human evolution. The sense of smell corresponds to the most ancient part of our history. Before being able to hear, see, and even think, beings felt and communicated by the sense of smell. When we humans were all still hunter-gatherers, this sense allowed us to identify an edible food or, to the contrary, protect us from danger.

Since the dawn of time and throughout evolution, each living species (animal or plant) has created defense mechanisms in a hostile environment. These defense mechanisms (which are determined genetically) are obviously fairly specific to species sharing the same biotope: we adjust in reaction to our hostile neighbor in order to survive.

This universal fight for survival has led and should lead again to the evolution of species.

Bibliography

Affoyon, Félix. 2010. *Les vrais mécanismes de la maladie d'Alzheimer et des maladies associées*. Dijon: François-Xavier de Guibert.

Alzheimer's Association. 2021. *2021 Alzheimer's Disease Facts and Figures*. Chicago: Alzheimer's Association.

Baltzer, Liana. 2016. "Olfaction et maladie d'Alzheimer: Une piste pour le diagnostic et le traitement?" Phd diss., University of Bordeaux.

Barnes, D. E., and K. Yaffe. 2011. "The Projected Effect of Risk Factor Reduction on Alzheimer's Disease Prevalence." *The Lancet Neurology* 10, no. 9: 819–28.

Bartczak, Sophie. 2015. "Les huiles essentielles réaniment l'hôpital." *Psychologies Magazine* (June): 174–78.

Besnault, Marion, and Miléna Thierry. 2016. "Apports des stimulations olfactives sur les représentations sémantiques des patients présentant une maladie d'Alzheimer." Master's thesis, Pierre and Marie Curie University (Paris).

Billioti de Gage, S., Y. Moride, T. Ducruet, T. Kurth, H. Verdoux, M. Tournier, et al. 2014. "Benzodiazepine Use and Risk of Alzheimer's Disease: Case-Control Study." *BMJ*: 349.

Bodin, Luc. 2007. *La maladie d'Alzheimer*. Paris: Éditions du Dauphin.

Bredesen, Dale. 2017. *The End of Alzheimer's*. New York: Avery.

Broom, G. M., I. C. Shaw, and J. J. Rucklidge. 2019. "The Ketogenic Diet as a Potential Treatment and Prevention Strategy for Alzheimer's Disease." *Nutrition* 60: 118–21.

Bushdid, C., M. O. Magnasco, L. B. Vosshall, and A. Keller. 2014. "Humans Can Discriminate More than 1 Trillion Olfactory Stimuli." *Science* 343, no. 6177: 1370–72.

Campbell, M. C. W., L. Emptage, F. Corapi, et al. 2017. "Amyloid Beta Deposits in Ex Vivo Retinas Correlate with the Severity of Alzheimer's Brain Pathology." *Investigative Ophthalmology & Visual Science* 58, no. 8: 1255.

Carmona-Gutierrez, D., A. Zimmermann, K. Kainz, F. Pietrocola, G. Chen, et al. 2019. "The Flavonoid 4,4'-dimethoxychalcone Promotes Autophagy-Dependent Longevity across Species." *Nature Communications* 10, no. 1: 651.

Chang, K. H., Y. C. Hsu, C. C. Hsu, C. L. Lin, C. Y. Hsu, C. Y. Lee, L. W. Chong, H. C. Liu, M. C. Lin, and C. H. Kao. 2016. "Prolong Exposure of NSAID in Patients with RA Will Decrease the Risk of Dementia: A Nationwide Population-Based Cohort Study." *Medicine* 95, no. 10: e3056.

Changeux, J.-P., P. Courrége, and A. Danchin. 1973. "A Theory of the Epigenesis of Neuronal Networks by Selective Stabilization of Synapses." *Proceedings of the National Academy of Sciences* 70, no. 10: 2974–78.

Chen, S. G., V. Stribinskis, M. J. Rane, et al. 2016. "Exposure to the Functional Bacterial Amyloid Protein Curli Enhances Alpha-Synuclein Aggregation in Aged Fischer 344 rats and *Caenorhabditis elegans*." *Scientific Reports* 6: 34477.

De Jesus Moreno Moreno, M. 2003. "Cognitive Improvement in Mild to Moderate Alzheimer's Dementia after Treatment with the Acetylcholine Precursor Choline Alfoscerate: A Multicenter, Double-Blind, Randomized, Placebo-Controlled Trial. *Clinical Therapeutics* 25, no. 1: 178–93.

de la Monte, S. M., and J. R. Wands. 2008. "Alzheimer's Disease Is Type 3 Diabetes: Evidence Reviewed." *Journal of Diabetes Science and Technology* 2, no. 6: 1101–13.

Dubois, B., J. Touchon, F. Portet, P. J. Ousset, B. Vellas, and B. Michel. 2002. "The '5 words': A Simple and Sensitive Test for the Diagnosis of Alzheimer's Disease. *Presse mèdicale* 31, no. 36: 1696–99.

Gaulier, Michel, and Marie-Thérèse Esneault. 2002. *Odeurs prisonnières*. Esqualquens: Éditions Quintessence.

Grosman, Marie, and Roger Lenglet. 2014. *Menace sur nos neurones: Alzheimer, Parkinson . . . et ceux qui en profitent*. Arles: Actes Sud.

Guo, H. D., J. Zhu, J. X. Tian, S. J. Shao, Y. W. Xu, et al. 2016.

"Electroacupuncture Improves Memory and Protects Neurons by Regulation of the Autophagy Pathway in a Rat Model of Alzheimer's Disease. *Acupuncture in Medicine* 34, no. 6: 449–56.

Hansson, O., H. Zetterberg, P. Buchhave, E. Londos, K. Blennow, and L. Minthon. 2006. "Association between CSF Biomarkers and Incipient Alzheimer's Disease in Patients with Mild Cognitive Impairment: A Follow-Up Study." *The Lancet Neurology* 5, no. 3: 228–34. Erratum in *The Lancet Neurology* 5, no. 4 (2006): 293.

Hofrichter, J., M. Krohn, T. Schumacher, C. Lange, B. Feistel, B. Walbroel, and J. Pahnke. 2016. "*Sideritis Spp.* Extracts Enhance Memory and Learning in Alzheimer's β-Amyloidosis Mouse Models and Aged C57B1/6 Mice." *Journal of Alzheimer's Disease* 53, no. 3: 967–80.

Huang, H. C., K. Xu, and Z. F. Jiang. 2012. "Curcumin-Mediated Neuroprotection against Amyloid-β-Induced Mitochondrial Dysfunction Involves the Inhibition of GSK-3β." *Journal of Alzheimer's Disease* 32, no. 4: 981–96.

Jimbo, D., Y. Kimura, M. Taniguchi, M. Inoue, and K. Urakami. 2009. "Effect of Aromatherapy on Patients with Alzheimer's Disease." *Psychogeriatrics* 9: 173–79.

Lambert, P. 2006. "La plasticité cérébrale." *Sciences Humaines,* no. 3. Updated July 6, 2015.

Laurin, D., R. Verreault, J. Lindsay, K. MacPherson, and K. Rockwood. 2001. "Physical Activity and Risk of Cognitive Impairment and Dementia in Elderly Persons." *Archives of Neurology* 58, no. 3: 498–504.

Lledo, Pierre-Marie. 2019. "Cette vieillesse pouvant devenir notre pire ennemie." *La Revue de la MTRL,* no. 101.

Lombion, S., L. Rumbach, and J. L. Millot. 2010. "Olfaction et pathologies neurodégénératives." *La Lettre du Neurologue,* no. 5.

Micas, Michèle. 2016. *Alzheimer.* Paris: Éditions Josette Lyon.

Montgomery, S. A., L. J. Thal, and R. Amrein. 2003. "Meta-Analysis of Double Blind Randomized Controlled Clinical Trials of Acetyl-L-Carnitine versus Placebo in the Treatment of Mild Cognitive Impairment and Mild Alzheimer's Disease." *International Clinical Psychopharmacology* 18, no. 2: 61–71.

Nehls, Michael. 2018. *Guérir Alzheimer.* Arles: Actes Sud.

Peyronnet, Mireille. 2010. *Prévenir Alzheimer*. Monaco: Alpen Éditions.

Podlesniy, P., J. Figueiro-Silva, A. Llado, et al. 2013. "Low Cerebrospinal Fluid Concentration of Mitochondrial DNA in Preclinical Alzheimer Disease. *Annals of Neurology* 74, no. 5: 655–58.

Polydor, Jean-Pierre. 2009. *Alzheimer, mode d'emploi*. Bordeaux: L'Esprit du Temps.

Rusek, M., R. Pluta, M. Ułamek-Kozioł, and S. J. Czuczwar. 2019. "Ketogenic Diet in Alzheimer's Disease. *International Journal of Molecular Sciences* 20, no. 16: 3892.

Saint-Jean, Olivier, and Éric Favereau. 2018. *Alzheimer, le grand leurre*. Paris: Éditions Michalon.

Schaal, Benoist, Thomas Hummel, and Robert Soussignan. 2004. "Olfaction in the Fetal and Premature Infant: Functional Status and Clinical Implications." *Clinics in Perinatology* 31: 261–85.

Selmès, Jacques, and Christian Derouesné. 2009. *La maladie d'Alzheimer pour les nuls*. Paris: First Éditions.

Serrand, Michèle. 2014. *Maladie d'Alzheimer, et s'il y avait un traitement?* Vergèze, France: Thierry Souccar Éditions.

Sohrabi, H. R., K. A. Bates, M. G. Weinborn, et al. 2012. "Olfactory Discrimination Predicts Cognitive Decline among Community-Dwelling Older Adults." *Translational Psychiatry* 2, no. 5: e118.

Stern, Y. 2017. "An Approach to Studying the Neural Correlates of Reserve." *Brain Imaging and Behavior* 11: 410–16.

Trivalle, Christophe. 2017. *101 conseils pour être bien dans son âge et dans sa tête*. Paris: Robert Laffont.

Yan, D., Y. Zhang, L. Liu, and H. Yan. 2016. "Pesticide Exposure and Risk of Alzheimer's Disease: A Systematic Review and Meta-Analysis." *Scientific Reports* 1, no. 6: 32222.

Index

acetylcholine, 58–59, 145, 188–90

acetyl-L-carnitine, 189–90

active depression, 78

adenosine triphosphate (ATP), 19–20, 21

Affoyon, Félix, 8–10

age, 97, 214

aging, 105

agitation, 76

air diffusers, 153–56

Air Synergy, 159

alpha-glyceryl-phosphoryl-choline, 189

aluminum, 91–92

Alzheimer, Alois, 14–15

Alzheimer's Association, 1

Alzheimer's dementia, 23–24

Alzheimer's disease. *See specific topics*

amino acids, 195–97

amygdala, 17

amyloid proteins, 18–19

anosmia, 7–8, 139

anticholinesterase drugs, 188

antioxidants, 20, 60

apathy, 78

aphasia, 73

APOE4 gene, 86

apolipoprotein (APOE), 37

application methods, 152–58

Aricept, 83

aromatic herbs, 177

arsenic, 94

ashitaba, 201

astrocytes, 120–21

atrophic causation, 4

attention, 25

autoimmune diseases, 110

autonomic nervous system, 13, 51

autophagy, 201–4

balance, 78

Baltzer, Liana, 38

Barnes, Deborah, 96

beans, 11–12

benzodiazepines, 82, 100–101

beta-amyloids, 3

biocides, 95

blood-brain barrier, 120–22

blood cells, 119

Bol d'air Jacquier, 197

brain, 51–52

   development of, 52–53

   hypovascularity of, 90

   oxygen for, 197–98

   structure of, 53–56

brain-intestines relationship, 115–16

brain training, 125

breath, 181

Bredesen, Dale, 4–5

Broca, Paul, 234

butterfly ginger, 146–47

cacosmia, 140

cadmium, 94–95

Canac, Patty, 13

cancer, 89, 110

cannabis, 102

canola oil, 90

cardiovascular disease, 89,
    98–99

caregivers, 205–13

care management, 211–12

cats, 233–34

causes of Alzheimer's disease
    AOPE4 gene, 86
    biocides and pesticides, 95
    heavy metals, 91–95
    hypovascularity of brain, 90
    as an iatrogenic disease, 81–83
    inflammation, 89–90
    mitochondria and, 84–86
    pathogenic track, 88–89

celiac disease, 107–8

cell phones, 103

cellular membrane, 19–20

cellular terrain, 217–18

central nervous system, 13, 51

cereal grains, 177

cerebral aging, 130–31

cerebral atrophy, 15

cerebral cortex, 55–56

cerebral hemispheres, 54

cerebral lesions, 14–15

cerebral reserve, 124

cerebral stimulants, 143–45

cerebrospinal fluid (CSF), 20, 35

Changeux, Jean-Pierre, 129

Chen, S. G., 19

chlorophyll, 11, 174

cholesterol, 98–99

chronos, 131–32

circulating immune complexes (CICs),
    121–22

citrus, 177

clary sage, 13

clock drawing test, 31–32

cognitive activity, 183–84

cognitive deficits, 70–71

cognitive functions, 29

cognitive reserves, 124–27

collagen, 119

communication, 206–7

compassion, 181

comprehension, 73

computed tomography (CT),
    33–34

condiments, 177

consolidation, 67

cooked food, 9–10

cooking, 163–70

copper:zinc ratio, 50

cortisol, 48

c-reactive protein (CRP), 44

cypress, 143–44

cytokines, 44–45

daily life, 2, 78
death, 211–13
defense mechanisms, 8
de la Monte, Suzanne, 87
delirious conviction, 76
delusional ideas, 75–76
dementia, defining, 22–24
depression, 78
DHA, 187
DHEA, 48
diabetes, 86–87, 105
diagnosis
    defining dementia, 22–24
    exam by general practitioner,
        27–28
    exams useful for, 29–36
    genetics and, 36–37
    multidisciplinary approach,
        26–27
    olfactory tests, 37–39
    specialists and, 28–29
diet, 96, 104–11
    amino acids, 195–97
    beneficial fatty acids, 186–87
    enzyme therapy, 198–99
    essential plants, 199–201
    modern, 85, 104–11
    raw foods, 8–9, 10, 171–78
    role of nutrition, 185–86
    vitamins, 190–93
dignity, 1
dogs, 228–34
donepezil, 83
dopamine, 58–59
dreams, 101–2

drugs, 102–3
DSM-V, 24

Earth Synergy, 160
education level, 97–98
elastic tissue, 119
electroacupuncture, 202
electromagnetic waves, 103–4
embryogenesis, 136
emotions, awakening, 128, 210
empathy, 209–10
encoding, 66
endocrine system, 13
End of Alzheimer's, The (Bredesen), 4
end-of-life distress, 152
environmental pollutants, 3
enzymatic processes, 10
enzymes, 165–66
enzyme therapy, 198–99
EPA, 187
essential oils
    application methods, 152–58
    choosing oils, 143–49
    effects of, 141–43
    olfactory testing with, 38–39
    stimulating sense of smell and, 12–13
    treating Alzheimer's with, 150–52
estrogen, 46–47
Eubiotic Synergy, 161
evening blends, 150–51
evolution, 5
explicit memory, 73

family members, 205–13
fatty acids, 186–87

fermented foods, 176–77
Fire Synergy, 160
first epoch: the raw, 8–9
First Forest Synergy, 161
fish, 90
five-word test, 31
flax, 90
flaxseed oil, 187
food. *See* cooking; diet
free radicals, 20, 85–86, 89
Free School of Natural and
    Ethnomedicine (FLMNE), 13
frontal lobe, 55
frontotemporal degenerations (FTD),
    219–22
fruit juice, 177–78
frying, 167–68
functional imaging, 32

GABA, 58–59, 145, 182
games, 184
gamma-oryzanol, 116
gender, 97
genetic risk, 7–8
genetics, 36–37
germinated seeds, 174–75
germs, 85
ginger, 13, 143–44
Ginkgo, 200
glucose, 86–87
glutathione, 116–17
gluten intolerance, 106–9
grains, 11–12
grains of paradise, 147
gray matter, 54

green juices, 11, 177–78
green tea, 200
grief, 212–13
grilling, 167–68

Hahnemann, Samuel, 217
hallucinations, 75, 224–25
Hatha yoga, 182
heavy metals, 91–95
herbe des rois, 147
high blood pressure, 98–99, 105
hippocampus, 16, 23, 53
Hippocrates, 5, 215
histamine, 49–50
homocysteine, 41
hormone status, 46–47
hospitals, 13, 142
human evolution, 5
hypermethylation, 50
hyperosmia, 139
hyposmia, 8, 139

incontinence, 79
inflammation, 3, 19, 89–90
inflammation markers, 43–45
inhalation, 152–53
insomnia, 152, 225
instinctotherapy, 173
insulin, 87
intellect, 78
intestinal barrier, 112–18
intestinal hyperpermeability, 109–10

Jacquier, René, 197
juice, 177–78

Kaqun Water, 198
katafray, 148
ketogenic diet, 87–88
kimchi, 176
Kouchakoff, Paul, 165
krill oil, 187
kryptopyrroles, 50

laboratory analysis
    detecting neurological or psychiatric
        disease, 49–50
    homocysteine, 41
    hormone status, 46–47
    inflammation markers, 43–45
    stress and, 47–48
    trace elements, 42–43
    vitamin D, 41–42
lactofermented vegetables, 176–77
Lambert, Philippe, 129
Lancet Neurology, 96
languages, 127
lavender, 13, 144–45
leaky gut syndrome, 82, 109–10
lesions, 117
leukocytosis, 165
Lewy body dementia, 223–26
L-glutamine, 116–17
life expectancy, 1
lifestyle changes, 4–5
limbic brain, 52–53
limbic system, 15–17
lipids, 167
lithium, 43, 194
living-food diet, 10–12
L-methione, 116

longevity, 216
long-term memory, 63–65
Lou Gehrig's disease, 122

macroscopic anomalies, 17–18
magnesium, 48
magnetic resonance imaging (MRI), 33
manavao, 148–49
marjoram, 144
massage, 156–58
medical history, 214–18
medications, 4, 81–83
meditation, 181
medium-chain triglycerides, 88
melancholy, 78
memorization, 66–67
memory, 61
    five systems of, 62–65
    neural network functioning, 65
    stages of, 65–68
memory loss, 1, 24, 68
memory's twilight, 72–73
mercury, 92–94
metabolism, 164–65
methionine, 197
microbiome, 113–14
microbiota, 18–19
microglial cells, 121
microwaves, 168–69
mild cognitive impairment, 24–26,
    69–70
mild stage, 71–72
minerals, 166
Mini-Mental State Examination
    (MMSE), 30–31, 70

mitochondria, 19–20, 84–86

mitochondrial alterations, 19–21

mobility, 79–80

moderate stage, 72–77

modern diet, 104–11

molecular imaging, 32–33

molecular mechanisms, 3–4

morning blends, 150

motivation, 25

motor behavior disturbances, 76–77

mountain tea, 201

muscle mass, 79–80

music, 180

Nehls, Michael, 216–17

neroli, 144, 151

nervous system disorders, 110

neural network functioning, 65

neurofibrillary degeneration, 17–18

neuroimaging, 32–34

neurologists, 28–29

neurometabolism, 49

neuronal signal transmission, 57–58

neuron capital, 58

neurons, 56–58

neuroplasticity
  awakening the brain in Alzheimer's patients, 127–29
  cognitive reserves, 123–27
  periods of brain development, 129–31
  time, 131–32

neuropsychological exam, 29–30

neurorestorative oils, 146–49

neuroscience, essential oils and, 12–13

neurotransmitters, 57–60, 187–90

NSAIDs, 90

nutrients, 165–67

nutrition, 185–86

nutritional deficiencies, 3

obesity, 89

Ohsumi, Yoshinori, 201

olfactory bulb, 53, 138

olfactory stress test, 39

olfactory system, 5–6, 138–40

olfactory tests, 37–39

olive oil, 90, 187

omega-3, 45, 90, 187

omega-6, 45, 90, 187

oral contraceptives, 122

orange zest, 13

organic diet, 96

organic silicon, 194

orientation, 74

oxidative stress, 21, 82, 85–86

oxygen, 90, 197–98

paleoanthropology, science of, 5

paleo lifestyle, 217

paleontology, 8–10

parchment paper, 170

parietal lobe, 55

Parkinson's disease, 122, 224

parosmia, 140

pathogens, 85, 88–89

patient's world, 206–11

peppermint, 13, 143–44

perceptive memory, 62–63

peripheral nervous system, 51

personality disorder, 2

pesticides, 89, 95

petitgrain, 13

phantosmia, 140

phenylalanine, 196

phosphatidylserine, 189

phosphorus, 21

phylogenesis, 8, 53

physical activity, 126–27, 183

Pick, Arnold, 223

Pick's disease, 223

plant-based diet, 11

Polydor, Jean-Pierre, 209–10, 211

positron emission tomography (PET), 34

potatoes, 11–12

prebiotics, 117–18

pregnenolone, 47

prevention, maintaining healthy mental state, 179–84

prevention policy, 6

probiotics, 117–18

procedural memory, 65

progesterone, 46–47

protective barriers

    blood-brain barrier, 120–22

    blood cells, 119

    intestinal barrier, 112–18

    reticuloendothelial system, 118–19

    vascular endothelium, 119

protein metabolism, 19–21

proteins, 166–67

Proust phenomenon, 64

psychotic disturbances, 74

Rabeau, Nelly, 162

raw foods, 8–9, 10, 171–78

reading, 184

reason, loss of, 1

reminiscence, 128

reptilian brain, 52

research, current state of, 2–5

restoration, 68

reticuloendothelial system, 118–19

retinal imaging, 35–36

risk factors

    age, 97

    cardiovascular factors, 98–99

    drugs, 102–3

    education level, 97–98

    electromagnetic waves, 103–4

    modern diet, 104–11

    sex, 97

    sleep, 100–102

    sleep apnea, 99–100

rosemary, 13, 143, 145

runaway episodes, 74

Saint-Jean, Oliver, 3

salt, 105–6

saro, 149

sauerkraut, 176

scent memory, 64

Schofield, Peter, 39

Schopenhauer, Arthur, 234

Sears, Robert W., 91

seaweeds, 177

second epoch: the cooked, 9–10

sedimentation rate, 43–45

seeds, 174–75

selenium, 42–43, 193

senile plaques, 17–18

senses, stimulating, 128–29

serotonin, 58–59

short-term memory, 63

silicon, 194

skull trauma, 98–99

sleep, 77, 100–102, 127

sleep apnea, 99–100

sleeping pills, 100–101

smell

    anatomical features involved in, 137–38

    dogs and, 228–34

    features of, 135–36

    loss of, 7–8

    memory of odors, 133–35

    science and, 235

social constructs, 3

social disease, 2

social networks, 125–26

speech, 73

spices, 177

spinal tap, 34–35

spirulina, 117

stages and progression

    cognitive defects as heart of disease, 70–71

    final stage, 79–80

    mild stage, 71–72

    moderate stage, 72–77

    onset of, 69

    severe stage, 77–79

steaming, 169–70

Stern, Yaakov, 124–25

storage, 66–67

stress, 47–48, 179

strokes, 23, 105

structural imaging, 32

subjective memory complaints, 24–25

sugar, 106

supplements, 116–17

surroundings, 74

systematic balance, 158–62

tau protein, 17, 18, 21

taurine, 196

temporal lobes, 15, 55

Thomas-Anterion, Catherine, 180

thyroid hormones, 46

time, 1, 74, 131–32

toxic causation, 4

toxins, 85

trace elements, 42–43, 193–94

triglycerides, 88

tryptophan, 196

turmeric, 116, 199

type 3 diabetes, 86–87

tyrosine, 195–96

understanding, 208–9

utero, in, 129–30

vaccines, 91–92, 93–94

validation therapy, 210

vascular dementia, 23, 227

vascular endothelium, 119

vegetable juice, 177–78

vegetables, 174

verbal memory, 16

violent behavior, 78–79
visual memory, 16
vitamin B, 50
vitamin D, 41–42, 204
vitamin E, 43
vitamins, 165, 190–93

walnut oil, 187
walnuts, 90
wandering, 74, 77
Water Synergy, 159
weight gain, 105
wheatgrass juice, 177–78
white matter, 54

Wi-Fi, 103
working memory, 63
World Health Organization,
    2–5
writing, 184

xenobiotics, 85

Yaffe, Kristine, 96
ylang-ylang, 13
yoga, 182–83

zinc, 42, 193–94
zinc citrate, 117